MILK CONSUMPTION

SELECT ANALYSES OF TRENDS AND VARIABLES

NUTRITION AND DIET RESEARCH PROGRESS

NUTRITION AND DIET RESEARCH PROGRESS

MILK CONSUMPTION

SELECT ANALYSES OF TRENDS AND VARIABLES

FRANCISCO PAUL BUREN

EDITOR

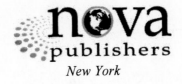

publishers

New York

For permission to use material from this book please contact us:
Telephone 631-231-7269; Fax 631-231-8175
Web Site: http://www.novapublishers.com

NOTICE TO THE READER

The Publisher has taken reasonable care in the preparation of this book, but makes no expressed or implied warranty of any kind and assumes no responsibility for any errors or omissions. No liability is assumed for incidental or consequential damages in connection with or arising out of information contained in this book. The Publisher shall not be liable for any special, consequential, or exemplary damages resulting, in whole or in part, from the readers' use of, or reliance upon, this material. Any parts of this book based on government reports are so indicated and copyright is claimed for those parts to the extent applicable to compilations of such works.

Independent verification should be sought for any data, advice or recommendations contained in this book. In addition, no responsibility is assumed by the publisher for any injury and/or damage to persons or property arising from any methods, products, instructions, ideas or otherwise contained in this publication.

This publication is designed to provide accurate and authoritative information with regard to the subject matter covered herein. It is sold with the clear understanding that the Publisher is not engaged in rendering legal or any other professional services. If legal or any other expert assistance is required, the services of a competent person should be sought. FROM A DECLARATION OF PARTICIPANTS JOINTLY ADOPTED BY A COMMITTEE OF THE AMERICAN BAR ASSOCIATION AND A COMMITTEE OF PUBLISHERS.

Additional color graphics may be available in the e-book version of this book.

Library of Congress Cataloging-in-Publication Data

ISBN: 978-1-62948-008-4

Published by Nova Science Publishers, Inc. † New York

CONTENTS

PREFACE

Most Americans do not consume enough dairy products. The Dietary Guidelines for Americans, 2010 recommends 2 cup-equivalents per day for children aged 2 to 3 years, 2.5 for those aged 4 to 8 years, and 3 for Americans older than age 8. However, per capita dairy consumption has long held steady at about 1.5 cup-equivalents, despite rising cheese consumption. This stasis in per capita dairy consumption results directly from the fact that Americans are drinking progressively less fluid milk. Since 1970 alone, per capita fluid milk consumption has fallen from 0.96 cup-equivalents to about 0.61 cup-equivalents per day. The Federal Government encourages dairy consumption, including fluid milk, cheese, and yogurt, among other foods, through the Dietary Guidelines for Americans, 2010. Special emphasis is placed on fat-free and low-fat products. USDA further supports this message through programs like the National School Lunch Program (NSLP). The NSLP stipulates that schools must provide fluid milk and it must be low-fat or skim, rather than whole. Dairy farmers and fluid milk processors are also working to promote dairy products. The popular "Got Milk?" campaign, for one, encourages drinking fluid milk. This book examines trends in Americans' fluid milk consumption including average portion sizes and generational differences in the frequency of milk drinking, to investigate possible explanations for the continued decreases.

Chapter 1 – Americans are drinking less fluid milk, on average. In this study, ERS researchers find that declining consumption since the 1970s reflects changes in the frequency of fluid milk intake, rather than changes in portions. USDA survey data collected between 1977 and 2008 reveal that Americans are less apt to drink fluid milk with their midday and nighttime meals than in earlier years, reducing the total number of consumption occasions per day. Moreover, more recent generations of Americans show greater decreases in consumption frequency, holding constant other factors such as education and race. The majority of Americans born in the 1990s consume fluid milk less often than those born in the 1970s, who, in turn, consume it less often than those born in the 1950s. All other factors constant, as newer generations with reduced demand gradually replace older ones, the population's average level of consumption of fluid milk may continue to decline.

Chapter 2 – Households have several ways to economize on their purchases at retail food stores when prices increase or their incomes fall. This report investigates a household's choice among retail fluid milk products categorized along three dimensions: three levels of fat content, two levels of package size, and organic versus conventional methods of production. Nielsen Homescan data from 2007-08 are used to estimate a choice model, which accounts for price, income, and other choice determinants. Results show that small changes in prices and income have a modest impact on a household's choice among milk products. However, households mitigate the impact of more substantial price and income shocks by switching from more expensive to less expensive products. The authors also find that the demand for organic milk is more sensitive to swings in income and food prices than is demand for conventional milk.

Chapter 3 – This report examines retail purchase data for 12 dairy products and margarine from the Nielsen 2007 Homescan data. Selected demographic and socioeconomic variables included in the Nielsen data are analyzed for their effects on aggregate demand and expenditure elasticities for the selected products. A censored demand system is used to derive the demand elasticities. The resulting estimates revealed that the magnitudes of 10 of the 13 own-price elasticities have absolute values greater than 1; substitute relationships are found among most dairy categories; expenditure elasticities are 1 or greater for 7 of the 13 products; and demographic and socioeconomic variables are statistically significant contributors to dairy demand.

Chapter 4 – Consumer interest in organic milk has burgeoned, resulting in rapid growth in retail sales of organic milk. New analysis of scanner data from 2004 finds that most purchasers of organic milk are White, high income, and well educated. The data indicate that organic milk carries the USDA organic seal about 60 percent of the time, most organic milk is sold in supermarkets, organic price premiums are large and vary by region, and most organic milk is branded.

In: Milk Consumption
Editor: Francisco Paul Buren

ISBN: 978-1-62948-008-4
© 2013 Nova Science Publishers, Inc.

Chapter 1

WHY ARE AMERICANS CONSUMING LESS FLUID MILK? A LOOK AT GENERATIONAL DIFFERENCES IN INTAKE FREQUENCY*

Hayden Stewart, Diansheng Dong and Andrea Carlson

ABSTRACT

Americans are drinking less fluid milk, on average. In this study, ERS researchers find that declining consumption since the 1970s reflects changes in the frequency of fluid milk intake, rather than changes in portions. USDA survey data collected between 1977 and 2008 reveal that Americans are less apt to drink fluid milk with their midday and night-time meals than in earlier years, reducing the total number of consumption occasions per day. Moreover, more recent generations of Americans show greater decreases in consumption frequency, holding constant other factors such as education and race. The majority of Americans born in the 1990s consume fluid milk less often than those born in the 1970s, who, in turn, consume it less often than those born in the 1950s. All other factors constant, as newer generations with reduced demand gradually replace older ones, the population's average level of consumption of fluid milk may continue to decline.

---

* This is an edited, reformatted and augmented version of the United States Department of Agriculture publication, Economic Research Report Number 149, dated May 2013.

Keywords: Fluid milk, fluid milk demand, fluid milk products, intake frequency, consumption frequency, generational change, cohort effects, portion sizes, milk drinking, dairy products, dairy checkoff, school lunches, consumer habits, childhood habits

WHAT IS THE ISSUE?

Most Americans do not consume enough dairy products. The *Dietary Guidelines for Americans, 2010* recommends 2 cup-equivalents per day for children aged 2 to 3 years, 2.5 for those aged 4 to 8 years, and 3 for Americans older than age 8. However, per capita dairy consumption has long held steady at about 1.5 cup-equivalents, despite rising cheese consumption. This stasis in per capita dairy consumption results directly from the fact that Americans are drinking progressively less fluid milk. Since 1970 alone, per capita fluid milk consumption has fallen from 0.96 cup-equivalents to about 0.61 cup-equivalents per day.

The Federal Government encourages dairy consumption, including fluid milk, cheese, and yogurt, among other foods, through the *Dietary Guidelines for Americans, 2010*. Special emphasis is placed on fat-free and low-fat products. USDA further supports this message through programs like the National School Lunch Program (NSLP). The NSLP stipulates that schools must provide fluid milk and it must be low-fat or skim, rather than whole. Dairy farmers and fluid milk processors are also working to promote dairy products. The popular "Got Milk?" campaign, for one, encourages drinking fluid milk.

This report examines trends in Americans' fluid milk consumption, including average portion sizes and generational differences in the frequency of milk drinking, to investigate possible explanations for the continued decreases.

WHAT DID THE STUDY FIND?

Data from USDA dietary intake surveys conducted between the 1970s and 2000s show that Americans—on occasions when they drink fluid milk—continue to consume about 1 cup (8 fluid ounces). Given the stability of portions, trends showing decreases in per capita consumption since the 1970s mainly reflect changes in consumption frequency. Between the 1970s and

2000s, people have become less apt to drink fluid milk at mealtimes, especially with midday and nighttime meals, reducing the total number of consumption occasions:

- Between surveys in 1977-78 and 2007-08, the share of preadolescent children who did not drink fluid milk on a given day rose from 12 percent to 24 percent, while the share that drank milk three or more times per day dropped from 31 to 18 percent.
- Between 1977-78 and 2007-08, the share of adolescents and adults who did not drink fluid milk on a given day rose from 41 percent to 54 percent, while the share that drank milk three or more times per day dropped from 13 to 4 percent.
- Underlying these decreases in consumption frequency are differences in the habit to drink milk between newer and older generations. All else constant (e.g., race and income), succeeding generations of Americans born after the 1930s have consumed fluid milk less often than their preceding generations:
- Americans born in the early 1960s consume fluid milk on 1.1 fewer occasions per day than those born before 1930.
- Americans born in the early 1980s consume fluid milk on 0.3 fewer occasions per day than those born in the early 1960s.

Differences across the generations in fluid milk intake may help account for the observed decreases in per capita fluid milk consumption in recent decades despite public and private sector efforts to stem the decline. Furthermore, these differences will likely make it difficult to reverse current consumption trends. In fact, as newer generations replace older ones, the population's average level of fluid milk consumption may continue to decline.

HOW WAS THE STUDY CONDUCTED?

ERS researchers pooled data from five USDA dietary intake surveys for analysis. These included the 1977-78 Nationwide Food Consumption Survey, the 1989-1991 Continuing Survey of Food Intakes by Individuals (CSFII), 1994-1996 CSFII, the 2003-04 National Health and Nutrition Examination Survey (NHANES), and the 2007-08 NHANES. Respondents in each survey were asked to report their intake of all foods and beverages on one or more days. This study focused on individuals' fluid milk consumption during a single, 24-hour period.

Researchers reviewed the existing literature on fluid milk demand, compared consumption data across periods in the different surveys, and then conducted a formal hypothesis test for whether newer generations are consuming fluid milk fewer times per day, and whether changes in portion sizes are also affecting consumption trends. This was accomplished by estimating an econometric model that predicts both the frequency and total quantity of fluid milk consumed by Americans who participated in USDA food consumption surveys, based on their birth year, race, household income, and demographic characteristics.

INTRODUCTION

Most Americans do not consume enough dairy products. The *Dietary Guidelines for Americans, 2010* recommends 2 cup-equivalents per day for children aged 2 to 3 years, 2.5 for those aged 4 to 8 years, and 3 for Americans older than age 8. By contrast, actual dairy consumption has held steady between 1.45 and 1.55 cup-equivalents per capita since the 1970s, despite a near tripling of cheese consumption over the past 40 years (USDA-ERS, 2013a). The reason for this stasis in overall dairy consumption is that Americans are drinking progressively less fluid milk.

Long a dietary staple, fluid milk once accounted for the majority of overall dairy consumption. However, as chronicled by Popkin (2010, p. 1), there has been a "slow continuous shift downward" in milk drinking since the 1940s. Since 1970 alone, per capita consumption has fallen from 0.96 to 0.61 cup-equivalents per day (USDA-ERS, 2013a). Moreover, this trend appears to cut across different age groups. Younger people aged 2 to 18 years consumed less fluid milk in the 2000s than did children and adolescents in the 1970s (Cavadini et al., 2000; Popkin, 2010).[1] Adults (over 18) have also been consuming less fluid milk over time (Enns et al., 1977; Popkin, 2010).

The Federal Government encourages dairy consumption, including fluid milk, cheese, and yogurt, among other products, through the *Dietary Guidelines for Americans, 2010*.[2] Special emphasis is placed on consuming more fat-free and low-fat milk and milk products in particular. These foods provide many of the same nutrients as higher fat dairy products with fewer calories (p. 38).

USDA further supports its dairy message through programs like the National School Lunch Program (NSLP), the Special Supplemental Nutrition Program for Women, Infants, and Children (WIC), and the Special Milk Program. The NSLP, for one, requires participating schools to offer students low-fat or skim fluid milk—and no whole milk. Only skim milk may be flavored (e.g., strawberry or chocolate).

Like the Federal Government, dairy farmers and fluid milk processors are concerned about low levels of dairy consumption. Both invest in checkoff[3] programs to increase sales of and demand for dairy products and ingredients (National Dairy Promotion and Research Board, 2013). Some efforts supported by checkoff programs focus primarily on fluid milk, including the popular "Got Milk?" campaign. Others like "Fuel Up to Play 60" emphasize all dairy products consumption, including milk drinking. This particular initiative encourages children to be physically active and "fuel up" with nutrient-rich foods like low-fat and skim milk, cheese, and yogurt. Dairy farmers contribute $0.15 per 100 pounds of milk they commercially market to checkoff programs, while fluid milk processors contribute $0.20 per 100 pounds they sell in consumer-type packages. Yet, so far, the efforts of dairy farmers, fluid milk processors, and the Federal Government have not increased dairy consumption to recommended levels, while fluid milk consumption continues to fall.

Previous research on declining fluid milk consumption—the main reason for stationary dairy consumption levels—finds that generational differences ("cohort effects") are a contributing factor. Using dietary intake surveys collected by USDA between the 1970s and the 2000s, Stewart et al. (2012) recently demonstrated that more recent generations consume smaller quantities of fluid milk. For example, on average, Americans born in the 1980s consume less fluid milk per day than Americans born in the 1960s, holding constant other factors such as income and race. These findings may reflect the persistence of childhood habits—each successive generation grows up less accustomed than their parents to drinking fluid milk and carries that habit forward into adult life.

In this study, ERS researchers used USDA dietary intake surveys from the 1970s, 1980s, 1990s, and 2000s to identify the number of times per day that Americans consume fluid milk, as well as to identify portion sizes. A possible explanation for decreases in the quantity of fluid milk consumed over time is that Americans are consuming it fewer times per day. However, Americans may also be using fluid milk in different ways. For example, if Americans consume fluid milk more often than they used to as a snack in a coffee drink and less often as a standalone beverage at mealtimes, then average portion sizes could change. Given Stewart et al.'s (2012) findings on generational change, the researchers also tested whether newer generations are consuming fluid milk less frequently than older generations.

IDENTIFYING TRENDS IN THE FREQUENCY AND QUANTITY OF FLUID MILK CONSUMPTION

To monitor trends in the American diet, ERS estimates the quantities of foods available for consumption annually (USDA-ERS, 2013b). ERS food availability data suggest that Americans have been consuming less fluid milk since the 1940s.

Data on per capita consumption since the 1970s (USDA-ERS, 2013a)[4] reveal a decrease in average consumption from about 0.96 cups to about 0.61 cups of fluid milk per day over the past 40 years (fig. 1). Increases in the consumption of 2-percent, 1-percent, and skim milk have partly offset decreases in whole milk consumption.[5] These products are hereafter referred to as *lower fat* milk. Consumption of lower fat milk products accounted for about 20 percent of total consumption in the 1970s and about 70 percent by the end of the 2000s.

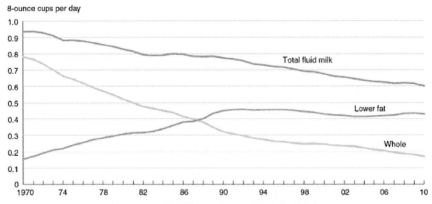

Source; Loss-Adjusted Food Availabilitym USDA ERS (2013a).
Notes: Whole milk has a fat of at least 3.25 perent, lower fat milk includes products
     with less milk fat than whole likw 2-perent, 1-percent, and skim milk.

Figure 1. Per capita, daily fluid, milk consumption declining.

Trends in fluid milk consumption can also be examined using USDA dietary surveys intermittently collected since the 1970s. Unlike ERS food availability data, these surveys break down food consumption data by particular segments of the population, such as children. Survey participants provided their household income, age, educational attainment, race, and ethnicity, among other characteristics. They also provided one or more 1-day "dietary recalls." These recalls include information on the foods and beverages consumed by the individual on the previous day.

The information provided shows how many times fluid milk was consumed, and whether each consumption occasion was part of a meal or snack. It is also possible to estimate the amounts of fluid milk consumed as a beverage, in cereal, or even as an ingredient in a food, such as a soup.[6] In this study, the researchers focused on individuals' fluid milk consumption over the 24-hour period covered by their initial 1-day dietary recall.

ERS limited the analysis to the consumption of plain and flavored fluid milk consumed alone as a beverage, put in cereal, poured in coffee, or used as an ingredient in selected coffee drinks.[7] In 2007-08, these products accounted for 93 percent of all fluid milk consumed by survey participants in all uses. Excluded from the study were milk in eggnog, malted milk, milkshakes, weight loss shakes, soups, and baked goods, among other foods. Also excluded from the results reported in this study were soy beverages.[8] USDA dietary records distinguish among whole, 2-percent, 1-percent, skim, and other types of fluid milk, though survey participants cannot always recall which type of milk they consumed. See also Appendix I: Comparing Consumption Across Different USDA Dietary Intake Surveys.

ERS analysis of USDA food consumption surveys collected since the 1970s confirms that fluid milk intake has declined for preadolescent children (aged 2 to 12 years), as well as for Americans beyond childhood (fig. 2). In 1977-78, preadolescent children drank, on average, 1.7 cups per day, while in 2007-08 children this age drank only 1.2 cups per day (30 percent less). Similarly, in 1977-78, Americans aged 13 and over drank, on average, 0.8 cups per day, while in 2007-08, people this age drank only 0.6 cups (25 percent less). USDA dietary intake surveys also confirm that milk drinkers in 2007-08 were more likely to choose a lower fat product than milk drinkers in 1977-78 (fig. 3).

To better understand declining fluid milk consumption, ERS examined how often Americans consume fluid milk at mealtimes (table 1). For example, in 1977-78, 39 percent of adolescents and adults drank milk with a morning meal; 24 percent consumed it with a midday meal; and 21 percent had fluid milk with a nighttime meal.[9] By 2007-08, those percentages had decreased to 28 percent, 8 percent, and 9 percent, respectively.

From the same two surveys, similar trends were seen in the consumption habits of preadolescent children. In the later survey, young children consumed fluid milk with fewer meals (especially, fewer midday and nighttime meals) than did the young children of the earlier survey. However, unlike adolescents and adults, young children have partly offset mealtime decreases in milk consumption with increases while snacking.

In total, Americans consumed fluid milk less frequently in 2007-08 than they did in 1977-78 or 1994-96 (fig. 4). Over the 30 years between 1977-78 and 2007-08, the share of individuals not consuming any fluid milk on a given day rose from 12 to 24 percent among preadolescent children, and from 41 to 54 percent among adolescents and adults. Furthermore, the shares consuming fluid milk several times a day fell. By 2007-08, only 45 percent of preadolescent children and 14 percent of adolescents and adults consumed fluid milk on more than one occasion.

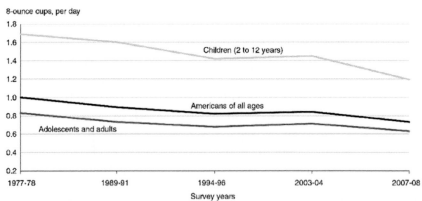

Source: Calculated by the authors using the 1977-78 Nationwide Food Consumption Survey (NFCS), 1989-1991 Continuing Survey of Food intakes by individuals (CSFII), 1994-1996 CSFII, 2003-04 National Health and Nutrition Examination Survey (NHANES), and 2007-08 NHANES and accompanying sample weights. Results are nased on all survey participants, including consumers who did not report consuming any fluid milk in their 1-day dietary recall.

Note: For all age categories shown above, daily per capita fluid milk consumption was lower in 1994-96 than in 1977-78. It was again lower in 2007-08 than in 1994-96. These differences are statistically significant at the 10-percent level.

Figure 2. Fluid milk consumption decreasing in all age groups.

Besides consuming milk less often, Americans may be changing their fluid milk-drinking habits in other ways, but so far, those changes have had little effect on portion sizes.

ERS researchers hypothesized that, if individuals are consuming fluid milk more often in a coffee beverage than they used to and less often as a standalone beverage at meals than they used to, average portion sizes may change.

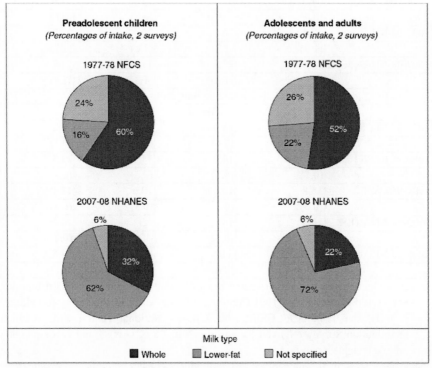

Source: Calculated by the authors using the 1977-78 Nationwide Food Consumption Survey (NFCS), 1989-1991 Continuing Survey of Food intakes by individuals (CSFII), 1994-1996 CSFLL, 2003-04 Nation Health and Nutrition Examination Survey (NHANES), and 2007-08 NHANES and accompanying sample weights.

Notes: Whole milk has a fat contents of at least 3.25 percent. Lower fat milk includes products with less milk fat than whole, like 2-percent, 1-percent, and skim milk. However, survey participants cannot always recall the fat content of milk they consumed. The type of milk is then "not specified".

Figure 3. Lower fat products now represent the bulk of fluid milk consumption for all age groups.

Table 1. Americans less apt to consume fluid milk at mealtimes[1]

Percentage of preadolescent children consuming fluid milk				
	Morning meal	Midday meal[2]	Night meal	Snack
1977-78 NFCS	71.3	50.7	35.5	19.9
	(0.6)	(0.7)	(0.7)	(0.5)
1989-91 CSFII	68.0	41.8	29.4	18.2
	(1.3)	(1.4)	(1.3)	(1.1)
1994-96 CSFII	64.0	33.7	23.5	21.0
	(0.9)	(0.9)	(0.8)	(0.8)
2003-04 NHANES	57.4	26.7	22.1	26.4
	(1.9)	(1.7)	(1.6)	(1.7)
2007-08 NHANES	55.6	29.3	17.5	24.7
	(1.7)	(1.5)	(1.3)	(1.4)
Percentage of adolescents and adults consuming fluid milk				
	Morning meal	Midday meal[2]	Night meal	Snack
1977-78 NFCS	38.8	24.0	21.5	13.2
	(0.4)	(0.4)	(0.3)	(0.3)
1989-91 CSFII	38.1	14.9	14.1	11.3
	(0.7)	(0.5)	(0.5)	(0.4)
1994-96 CSFII	35.8	10.4	10.6	12.1
	(0.6)	(0.4)	(0.3)	(0.4)
2003-04 NHANES	28.9	7.4	9.3	14.4
	(0.9)	(0.5)	(0.6)	(0.7)
2007-08 NHANES	28.2	8.0	8.8	13.8
	(0.8)	(0.5)	(0.6)	(0.7)

Source: Calculated by the authors using the 1977-78 Nationwide Food Consumption Survey (NFCS), the 1989-1991 Continuing Survey of Food Intakes by Individuals (CSFII), the 1994-1996 CSFII, the 2003-04 National Health and Nutrition Examination Survey (NHANES), and the 2007-08 NHANES and accompanying sample weights.

Notes: Decreases in the percentages of individuals consuming fluid milk with their morning, midday, and nighttime meals between 1977-78 and 2007-08 are statistically significant at the 10-percent level for both age groups.

[1]Standard errors reported in parentheses.

[2]Midday meal is defined as a meal occasion occurring between 11 a.m. and 5 p.m.

Nonetheless, from the data available, ERS finds that, on the occasions when Americans do consume fluid milk, they have continued to drink at least as much as they did in the 1970s (fig. 5). Americans drank about 1 cup (8 fluid ounces) of fluid milk per occasion in 2007-08, on average, versus 0.8 cups in 1977-78. That portions appear not to have decreased, in turn, suggests that decreases in the frequency of consumption, shown in table 1 and figure 4, primarily underlie the downward trend in intake, shown in figures 1 and 2.

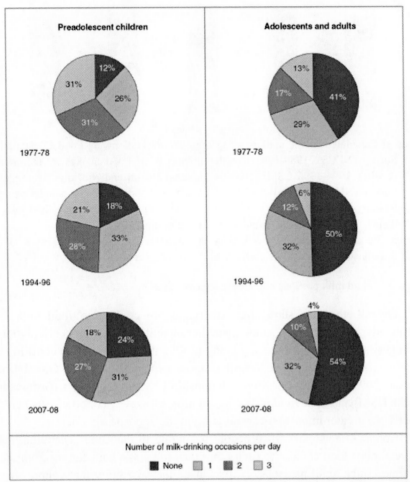

Figure 4. Americans consume fluid milk less frequently per day.

Source: Calculated by the authors using the 1977-78 Nationwide Food Consumption Survey (NFCS), 1989-1991 Continuing Survey of Food Intakes by Individuals (CSFII),1994-1996 CSFII, 2003-04 National Health and Nutrition Examination Survey (NHANES), and 2007-08 NHANES and accompanying sample weights.

Notes: Notable changes from the older to the newer surveys include increases in the percentages of individuals reporting no fluid milk consumption, as well as decreases in the percentages who consumed fluid milk on three or more occasions. These changes are statistically significant at the 10-percent level.

Figure 4.Americans consume fluid milk less frequently per day.

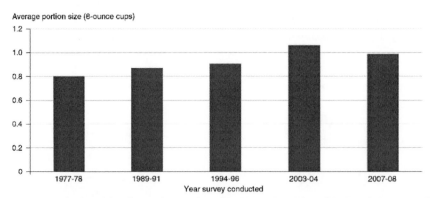

Average portion size (8-ounce cups)

Source: Calculated by the authors using the 1977-78 Nationwide Food Consumption Survey (NFCS), 1989-1991 Continuing Survey of Food intakes by individuals (CSFII), 1994-1996 CSFII, 2003-04 National Health and Nutrition Examination Survey (NHANES), and 2007-08 NHANES and accompanying sample weights. Results are based on survey participants, who reported consuming fluid milk in their 1-day dietary recall, excluding all nonconsumers.

Note: The average portion was largest in 2003-04 and sallest in 1977-78. Thiss difference is statistically significant at the 10-percent level.

Figure 5. Fluid milk portions not decreasing over time.

Overall, the data show that Americans are consuming fluid milk less frequently and, in turn, consuming smaller quantities, but what is driving these changes in behavior? Kaiser and Dong (2006) and Kaiser (2010) confirm that promotions sponsored by checkoff programs increase demand. Gleason and Suitor (2001) confirm a positive relationship between children's participation in the NSLP and their fluid milk consumption. However, cohort effects may be exerting a greater impact on consumption in the opposite direction.

Cohort effects exist when people belonging to the same generation make more similar food choices to each other than to people born farther from them in time. Since Schrimper (1979) first raised the possibility that cohort effects exist and shape trends in food consumption, much empirical research has followed. Mori et al. (2006) and Mori and Saegusa (2010) find that cohort effects influence fresh fruit and fish consumption in Japan. Stewart and Blisard (2008) find that they influence expenditures on fresh vegetables for at-home consumption in the United States.

As to cohort effects and fluid milk consumption, Stewart et al. (2012) find that more recent generations of Americans drink less fluid milk. For example, Americans born in the 1960s are consuming 0.13 cups less whole milk and 0.28 cups less lower fat milk per day than Americans born before 1930, holding constant other factors like race and income. Moreover, Americans born in the 1980s consume 0.16 cups less whole milk and 0.13 cups less lower fat milk per day than those born in the 1960s.

Cohort effects could influence U.S. fluid milk consumption for several reasons. These reasons begin with the unique experiences of each generation of American children. Every decade brings a wider selection of beverage choices at supermarkets, restaurants, and other food outlets. Soft drinks, isotonic sports drinks, bottled water, and other products increasingly compete with fluid milk for a share of the consumer's appetite. Changes have also occurred over time in the popularity of fast food, among other phenomena.

Changes in the food environment can affect children's beverage consumption. Fisher et al. (2001) and Bowman et al. (2004) suggest that children's fluid milk consumption may decrease with exposure to competing beverages and fast food, respectively. Regardless of other reasons, as successive generations of Americans have grown up amid declining rates of fluid milk consumption, they may have developed different life-long habits. The habit to drink milk may form (or not form) in childhood. According to the *Dietary Guidelines for Americans, 2010*, individuals "who consume milk at an early age are more likely to do so as adults" (p. 38).

MODELING TRENDS IN FLUID MILK CONSUMPTION ACROSS THE GENERATIONS

Investigating consumption differences over time and across generations requires a particular type of data set. Many studies of U.S. food demand use time series data. These data typically span several decades and include information on food consumption or expenditures, price, and consumer income. However, time series data also tend to be highly aggregated. They do not typically contain information on individual consumers. By contrast, cross-sectional data contain information on individual consumers and may, therefore, be suitable for investigating the effects of demographic characteristics on demand. Nonetheless, because such data seldom span more than a couple years, they are not ideal for studying longrun trends. In Deaton's (1997) terminology, researchers need a "time series of cross sections." That is, they must pool cross-sectional surveys collected over several decades. Mori and Stewart (2011) empirically demonstrate the advantages of such data over traditional time series data. In this study, ERS pools the 1977-78 Nationwide

Food Consumption Survey (NFCS), 1989-1991 Continuing Survey of Food Intakes by Individuals (CSFII), 1994-1996 CSFII, 2003-04 National Health and Nutrition Examination Survey (NHANES), and 2007-08 NHANES.

A time series of cross-sectional surveys provides information on each generation's food choices at various times in history and at different ages in their lives. For example, ERS researchers observed the number of times per day that members of different generations reported consuming fluid milk in the 1977-78 NFCS and in the 2007-08 NHANES (fig. 6). As young children in 1977-78, Americans born in the 1970s tended to consume fluid milk almost twice a day; and by 2007-08, as young adults in their 20s or 30s, they consumed it only 0.56 times per day. Despite their youth, Americans born in the 1970s consumed fluid milk even less often in 2007-08 than members of some older generations. Over a 30-year span, Americans born in the 1940s decreased the frequency of their fluid milk consumption from about 0.97 times per day (in 1977-78, in their 20s or 30s) to about 0.71 times per day (in 2007-08, in their 50s or 60s).

Previous studies, including Popkin (2010), Cavadini et al. (2000), and Stewart et al. (2012), have examined trends in the level of U.S. per capita fluid milk consumption. In this study, ERS researchers further investigated whether the smaller quantities of fluid milk being consumed by Americans are a result of their consuming it fewer times throughout the day. The researchers also confirmed whether trends in portion sizes likewise affect consumption levels. This was accomplished by estimating an econometric model that predicts both the frequency and total quantity of fluid milk consumed by Americans based on their generation (decade of birth), incomes, and demographic characteristics. Definitions and mean values are provided in table 2 for the model's dependent and explanatory variables. In the next section, these variables are explained and the model outlined.

Variables Used in the Analysis

The analysis focuses on fluid milk consumption by USDA survey participants over 24 hours. The number of times that an individual drank fluid milk during this period is denoted as FREQUENCY. Preadolescent children consumed fluid milk on 1.65 occasions, on average, with moderate person-to-person variation. FREQUENCY had a standard deviation of 1.2, among preadolescent children. By contrast, adolescents and adults consumed fluid milk 0.81 times, on average, with a standard deviation of 1.01.

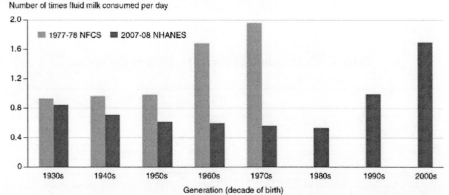

Source: Calculated by the authors using the 1977-78 Nationwide Food Consumption Survey (NFCS) and 2007-08 national Health and Nutrition Examination Survey (NHANES) and accompanying sample weights.Results are based on all survey participants, including those who did not report consuming any fluid milk in their 1-day dietary recall.

Note: Statistically significant \differences at the 10-percent level between the generations include those between Americans born in the 1940s and Americans born in the 1970s both in 1977-78 and 2007-08.

Figure 6. Frequency of fluid milk intake for different generations at different points in time.

Of all survey participants, 58 consumed fluid milk on more than 6 occasions. Three people consumed it on more than 10 occasions. The maximum value of FREQUENCY was 16 occasions.

Also of interest was a survey participant's total consumption of fluid milk. This dependent variable is denoted as QUANTITY. During the 24 hours covered by the dietary recall of preadolescent children, the children—including those who consumed no fluid milk at all—reported consuming 1.48 cups of fluid milk, on average, over all consumption occasions. Adolescents and adults consumed a total of 0.71 cups, on average. On the occasions when Americans do drink fluid milk, they may consume it in portions that are about what they were in the 1970s (see fig. 5). If portions have changed little, then changes over time in QUANTITY may reflect primarily changes in FREQUENCY.

The researchers also created explanatory variables to proxy for exogenousfactors that may influence a person's demand for fluid milk. FREQUENCY and QUANTITY were hypothesized to vary with a person's income, demographic characteristics, and his or her decade of birth, among other factors.

Table 2. Mean values of variables used in the model

		Children (age 2-12)	Adolescents and adults
FREQUENCY	Number of times fluid milk was consumed	1.65	0.81
QUANTITY	Total intake of fluid milk over 24 hours (cups)	1.48	0.71
INCOME	Household income (per capita 2003 dollars)	10,893.84	18,282.27
AGE	Age at the time of survey participation (years)	6.96	42.21
HHSIZE	Number of people living in household	4.52	3.13
PREGNANT	1 for pregnant; 0 otherwise		0.01
DIETING	1 for on a special diet; 0 otherwise		0.07
HISPANIC	1 for Hispanic ethnicity; 0 otherwise	0.14	0.09
BLACK	1 for Black; 0 otherwise	0.15	0.11
MALE	1 for male; 0 otherwise	0.51	0.46
COLLEGE	1 if household head finished college; 0 otherwise	0.28	0.29
WEEKEND	1 if dietary recall for a weekend; 0 otherwise	0.25	0.26
C1	1 if born prior to 1930; 0 otherwise		0.17
C2	1 if born between 1930-1934; 0 otherwise		0.05
C3	1 if born between 1935-1939; 0 otherwise		0.05
C4	1 if born between 1940-1944; 0 otherwise		0.07
C5	1 if born between 1945-1949; 0 otherwise		0.08
C6	1 if born between 1950-1954; 0 otherwise		0.09
C7	1 if born between 1955-1959; 0 otherwise		0.10
C8	1 if born between 1960-1964; 0 otherwise		0.11
C9	1 if born between 1965-1969; 0 otherwise		0.07
C10	1 if born between 1970-1974; 0 otherwise		0.07
C11	1 if born between 1975-1979; 0 otherwise		0.06
C12	1 if born between 1980-1984; 0 otherwise		0.04
C13	1 if born between 1985-1989; 0 otherwise		0.03
C14	1 if born between 1990-1994; 0 otherwise		0.02
TIME1	1 if 1977-78 NFCS; 0 otherwise	0.17	0.16
TIME2	1 if 1989-91 CSFII; 0 otherwise	0.21	0.20
TIME3	1 if 1994-96 CSFII; 0 otherwise	0.37	0.35
TIME4	1 if 2003-04 NHANES; 0 otherwise	0.13	0.14
TIME5	1 if 2007-08 NHANES; 0 otherwise	0.13	0.15

Source: Calculated by the authors using the 1977-78 Nationwide Food Consumption Survey (NFCS), the 1989-1991 Continuing Survey of Food Intakes by Individuals (CSFII), the 1994-1996 CSFII, the 2003-04 National Health and Nutrition Examination Survey (NHANES), and the 2007-08 NHANES and accompanying sample weights.

Extensive research has been conducted on methods for specifying this type of model. In this study, ERS followed procedures outlined by Deaton (1997), Johnson (1980), and Stewart and Blisard (2008) for defining explanatory variables and identifying cohort effects.

Previous studies have analyzed the effects of income, age, gender, race, ethnicity, and other demographic characteristics on fluid milk consumption. Based on Lin et al. (2003) and Davis et al. (2010), among other papers cited in this study, researchers defined several variables for inclusion in the model (table 2). These included the natural logarithm of a person's age (AGE), which is consistent with research showing that fluid milk consumption tends to be stable in childhood, falls in adolescence, and continues to fall at a slower rate throughout adulthood (e.g., Lin et al., 2003; Mannino et al., 2004; Sebastian et al., 2010). The researchers also included the natural logarithms of a person's household income (INCOME) and household size (HHSIZE), as well as binary variables for gender (MALE), race (BLACK), ethnicity (HISPANIC), whether at least one head of household has completed college (COLLEGE), and whether consumption was reported for a Saturday or Sunday (WEEKEND). For teenagers and adults, the researchers added binary variables to control for whether survey participants were dieting (DIETING) or pregnant (PREGNANT) during the 24 hours described in their 1-day dietary recall.

In addition to factors identified as important determinants of fluid milk consumption in past studies, researchers included explanatory variables for testing whether the number of times per day that a person consumes fluid milk varies across the generations. These binary explanatory variables include C2, for people born 1930- 34; C3, 1935-39; and so on in 5-year intervals, up to C14, 1990-94. By including C2 through C14 in the econometric model, the researchers could calculate the expected differences in consumption between each of these more recent cohorts and Americans born prior to 1930.[10] Evidence that more recently born cohorts consume fluid milk less often than older cohorts would confirm that a cohort effect is contributing to declining consumption frequency. By contrast, finding no consistent variance of consumption frequency across generations would refute the hypothesis that cohort effects are part of the trend.

ERS researchers also created binary variables that identify which USDA survey an individual joined. One of these binary variables, TIME2, indicates that an individual participated in the 1989-91 CSFII. Likewise, TIME3 identifies participants in the 1994-96 CSFII. And, finally, TIME4 and TIME5 denote participants in the 2003-04 and the 2007-08 NHANES. The estimation results on these four variables compare participants in the 1977-78 NFCS with participants in each of the subsequent surveys, holding all other explanatory variables in the model constant.[11] Unlike C2 through C14, which capture differences between the generations likely related to their experiences as children, TIME2 through TIME5 were hypothesized to capture the contemporaneous effects on all individuals of the availability of competing beverages and other aspects of the food marketing system.

Finally, ERS created a variable to account for prices. Prices for fluid milk have tended to fluctuate relative to prices for other nonalcoholic beverages. The researchers divided the Consumer Price Index (CPI) for fresh whole milk by the CPI for all nonalcoholic beverages.[12] The ratio of the two CPIs was 0.98 in 1977, 1.03 in 1989, 1.04 in 1994, 1.16 in 2003, and 1.34 in 2007. Values greater than one indicate that the cost of fresh whole milk has increased faster than the cost of nonalcoholic beverages in general. However, the inclusion of the price variable in addition to TIME2 through TIME5 did not improve estimation results. The likely reason is that, as compared with data in a typical time series study, the available data showed the food choices of Americans at only a small number of different price levels. Although the USDA dietary surveys pooled for this study collectively span over 30 years, data were available only for the years in which one of the five surveys was administered. Thus, the price variable was excluded from the final model.

Model Specification

How many times per day will an individual consume fluid milk products? The dependent variable FREQUENCY takes on only integer values: zero for nonconsumers, 1 for single occasion consumers, 2 for those who consumed on two occasions, and so on. Econometric models optimized for analyzing this type of data include the Poisson and negative binomial regression models. Greene (1997) provides a technical overview of each. Dong et al. (2000) used these models to study the number of times individuals patronize a restaurant. He et al. (2004) used the negative binomial model to analyze the number of times people consume beef, poultry, and seafood. In this study, ERS researchers assumed that the number of times a person drinks fluid milk could be approximated by the outcome of a Poisson distribution. By this model, the predicted value (conditional mean) of FREQUENCY is $\ddot{e} = e\hat{a}^X$ where e is the base of the natural logarithm, X is a set of explanatory variables, and $\hat{a}$ includes the parameters that describe the relationship between the dependent and explanatory variables by their sign (+/-) and magnitude. The researchers included in X a person's income, demographic characteristics, decade of birth, and survey year. Of course, the number of times that a particular individual consumes fluid milk may vary from the predicted value on any given day. The Poisson regression model assumes that the mean and variance of FREQUENCY conditional on X are the same. Both equal ë. However, the closely related negative binomial regression model relaxes this assumption. It instead assumes that FREQUENCY has conditional mean ë and conditional variance ë(1 + (1/è)ë) where 1/è is an "overdispersion" parameter. Thus, the conditional variance of FREQUENCY may exceed its conditional mean because of either heterogeneity across survey participants or omission from the regression model of demand determinants for which the necessary data do not exist to explicitly create explanatory variables. Researchers who work with count data will commonly estimate both a Poisson and negative binomial model. They then select between the two specifications by conducting a test for overdispersion.

The model further adds a second equation to the basic count data model for a survey participant's total daily intake of fluid milk over all consumption occasions. The value of QUANTITY is zero if FREQUENCY equals zero (i.e., for consumers who drank no milk). For other consumers, QUANTITY = aZ, where Z is a set of explanatory variables and a contains the parameters that describe the relationship among the variables. Researchers hypothesized that QUANTITY depends partly on the number of times a person consumed fluid milk. Thus, FREQUENCY is included in Z, along with the demographic characteristics of an individual that may influence portion sizes, such as his or her gender and age. Finally, the four survey date variables are included in Z. If the parameters on TIME2 through TIME5 are found to be negative and increasingly large in magnitude from older to newer surveys, then that would suggest that portion sizes have tended to decrease since the 1970s. Otherwise, it can be concluded that changing portion sizes have not contributed much to the decline in fluid milk consumption shown in figures 1 and 2.

The two-equation model in this study is a triangular system. FREQUENCY is modeled in the first equation and, in turn, helps to determine the value of QUANTITY in the second equation. However, in this type of model, biased estimates of the relationship between FREQUENCY and QUANTITY may result if FREQUENCY is simply included among the other explanatory variables in Z in our second equation.[13] To mitigate this problem, ERS researchers instead included the number of times per day that an individual is predicted to consume fluid milk, $ë=e^{ax}$, in Z.[14]

The researchers also allowed for the possibility that different factors may influence the food choices of preadolescent children and Americans age 13 and older. The two-equation model is estimated separately for people in these two age groups. Excluded from the model for preadolescent children are C2 through C14, PREGNANT, and DIETING. C2 through C14 are excluded from this model because it is customary to assume that young children are free of any habits associated with their year of birth (e.g., Mori and Saegusa, 2010); rather, they are still forming the habits that will later define their generation.

Estimation of the model in the present study makes a novel contribution to research on fluid milk consumption and the broader body of research on food demand. In contrast to previous studies of milk demand like Lin et al. (2003) and Davis et al. (2010) that use cross-sectional data, this study instead pools surveys collected over 30 years.

Moreover, to the authors' knowledge, this study represents the first application of count models to pooled survey data for testing whether generational change contributes to trends in the consumption of any food commodity. Additional information on the model, including the complete likelihood function, is provided in Appendix II: Model Specification and Estimation.

ESTIMATING THE MODEL AND EXAMINING RESULTS

Using data from the pooled USDA food consumption surveys, researchers estimated both the model for preadolescent children and the model for Americans beyond their preadolescent years by weighted maximum likelihood.[15]

As a preliminary exercise, the researchers initially estimated only the first equation for FREQUENCY as a standalone model. Poisson and negative binomial specifications were both considered. The researchers then used tests for overdispersion to select between these two specifications. Based on these test results, the researchers selected a Poisson model for preadolescent children and a negative binomial model for teenagers and adults.[16] The complete models, including the second equation for QUANTITY, were then estimated. The standard errors of $\hat{a}$ and $\hat{a}$ were calculated using a bootstrap procedure.[17] Lastly, ERS researchers confirmed the robustness of their key results.[18] The results of model estimation are reported in table 3 and table 4. As a supplementary exercise, the researchers used these results to predict how a change in each of the birth year (C2 through C14) and time variables

(TIME2 through TIME5) would affect the number of times per day that a person consumes fluid milk products (FREQUENCY).[19] These marginal effects are shown in figures 7 and 8.

Table 3. Frequency and quantity of fluid milk consumption, coefficient estimates for adolescents and adults

	FREQUENCY		QUANTITY	
Coefficient		Std. Error	Coefficient	Std. Error
Birth year (generation) variables				
C2	-0.31*	0.03		
C3	-0.48*	0.03		
C4	-0.60*	0.03		
C5	-0.64*	0.04		
C6	-0.82*	0.04		
C7	-0.92*	0.04		
C8	-0.90*	0.05		
C9	-1.21*	0.05		
C10	-1.28*	0.06		
C11	-1.30*	0.07		
C12	-1.35*	0.08		
C13	-1.47*	0.09		
C14	-1.42*	0.10		
Time (survey) variables				
TIME2	0.04	0.02	0.05	0.03
TIME3	0.04	0.02	0.04	0.03
TIME4	0.05	0.03	0.27*	0.04
TIME5	0.10*	0.04	0.10	0.04
Income and demographic variables				
ln(INCOME)	-0.03*	0.01	-0.02*	0.01
ln(AGE)	-0.70*	0.04	-0.52*	0.02
ln(HHS)	0.04*	0.01		
MALE	0.05*	0.01	0.39*	0.01
WEEKEND	-0.12*	0.01		
COLLEGE	0.09*	0.01	-0.05*	0.02
PREGNANT	0.44*	0.04	0.39*	0.06
DIETING	-0.04	0.02	-0.07	0.03
BLACK	-0.55*	0.02	-0.14*	0.03
HISPANIC	-0.04	0.02	-0.19*	0.02
Other model parameters				
CONSTANT	3.27*	0.18	3.13*	0.11
1/è	0.22*	0.01		
λ			0.17*	0.06

* = significant at the 1-percent level.

Source: Model estimated by ERS researchers using weighted maximum likelihood, sample weights provided by data in the 1977-78 Nationwide Food Consumption Survey (NFCS), the 1989-1991 Continuing Survey of Food Intakes by Individuals (CSFII), the 1994-1996 CSFII, the 2003-04 National Health and Nutrition Examination Survey (NHANES), and the 2007-08 NHANES. Standard error of equation for QUANTITY was 1.2.

Generational Change Contributing to Decreases in Frequency of Consumption

The results confirm that newer generations of Americans are consuming fluid milk products fewer times per day. For adolescents and adults, the marginal effects of the birth year variables represent the expected differences in consumption between a person born before 1930 and one born more recently, all else constant. For example, Americans born in the early 1960s are expected to consume fluid milk on about 1.1 fewer occasions per day at age 20, age 30, and so on than Americans born before 1930 consume at each of these same ages. This marginal effect is calculated using the estimation results for C8 (fig. 7).

Moreover, Americans born in the early 1980s are expected to consume fluid milk on about 0.3 occasions less per day than those born in the early 1960s. This finding follows from the estimation result for C8 and C12 and is also depicted in figure 7. Such large decreases in the frequency of consumption between individuals born several decades apart could gradually reduce per capita consumption as successively newer generations slowly replace older generations and account for a steadily larger share of the overall population.

If there were no cohort effect and the other explanatory variables in the model had remained unchanged, American adolescents and adults would have likely maintained the frequency of their fluid milk consumption from the 1970s into the 2000s. This conclusion follows from the marginal effects of TIME2 through TIME5 (fig. 8).

As discussed above, these variables are hypothesized to capture the contemporaneous effects of the food marketing system such as the availability of competing beverages. For adolescents and adults, these effects are small and do not tend to increase or decrease in magnitude from the older to more recent USDA food consumption surveys. Once people are past childhood, their food choices seem to be much more influenced by their childhood-formed habits than by changes over their life times in the environment in which their food choices are made.

However, changes over time in the food environment—that is, trends in prices, mix of competing products, etc.—appear responsible for reducing children's fluid milk consumption. As also shown in figure 8, these effects are increasingly negative from the older to the newer surveys for preadolescent children. We find that preadolescent children tended to drink milk on 0.28 fewer occasions per day in 1994-96 than did preadolescent children in 1977-

78, all else constant. By 2007-08, they were consuming it on 0.42 fewer occasions per day than in 1977-78.

Table 4. Frequency and quantity of fluid milk consumption, coefficient estimates for preadolescent children

	FREQUENCY		QUANTITY	
	Coefficient	Std. Error	Coefficient	Std. Error
Time (survey) variables				
TIME2	-0.10*	0.02	0.00	0.04
TIME3	-0.16*	0.02	-0.10*	0.04
TIME4	-0.19*	0.03	0.03	0.05
TIME5	-0.25*	0.02	-0.22*	0.05
Income and Demographic variables				
ln(INCOME)	-0.04*	0.01	-0.02	0.01
ln(AGE)	-0.19*	0.01	0.18*	0.03
ln(HHS)	0.02	0.03		
MALE	0.05*	0.01	0.19*	0.02
WEEKEND	-0.22*	0.02		
COLLEGE	0.08*	0.02	0.01	0.03
BLACK	-0.32*	0.02	-0.19*	0.05
HISPANIC	-0.01	0.02	0.06	0.03
Other model parameters				
CONSTANT	1.37*	0.11	1.18*	0.27
λ			0.30*	0.08

* = significant at the 1-percent level.

Source: Model estimated by ERS researchers using weighted maximum likelihood, sample weights provided by data in the 1977-78 Nationwide Food Consumption Survey (NFCS), the 1989-1991 Continuing Survey of Food Intakes by Individuals (CSFII), the 1994-1996 CSFII, the 2003-04 National Health and Nutrition Examination Survey (NHANES), and the 2007-08 NHANES. Standard error of equation for QUANTITY was 1.12.

Finally, the estimation results for household income and demographic variables generally agree with past studies. As shown in table 3, Americans drink milk fewer times per day as they age.

Change in number of times fluid milk consumed per day

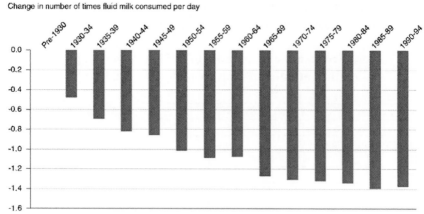

Approximate year of birth

Source: Marginal effects calculated by ERS researchers. Using standard techniques for nonlinear models, ERS researchers calculated the marginal effects from data in the 1077-78 nationwide Food Consumption Survey (NFCS), the 1989-1991 Continuing Survey of Food intakes by individuals (CSFII), the 1994-1996 CSFII, the 2003-04 National Health and Nutrition Examination Survey (NHANES), and the 2007-08 NHANES.

Notes: Estimated model for FREQUENCY used to calculate marginal effect. In the first step, ERS used to estimated model to predict the number of times per day that each adolescent and adult in the sample would have consumed fluid milk, of he or she had been born prior to 1930. All birth year variables. C2 though C14, were set equal to zero for this simulation. In the second step, the researchers re-predicted the value of FREQUENCY for each individuals once for each of 13 alternative scenarios: if the survey participant had instead been born from 1930 to 1934 (only C2 equals one), from 1935 to 1939 (only C3 equals to one), and so on. Finally the first-step results were subtracte from the second-step results. Marginal effects equal the average differences in the predicted value of COUNT, if individuals had been born prior to 1930 versus having been born during each of these subsequent time intervals, weighted by the sample weight. All effects are statistically significant at the 1-percent level.

Figure 7. Marginal effect of birth cohort on fluid milk consumption, adolescents and adults.

They also consume it more frequently if at least one head of household has completed college. From these results and the findings of existing studies, it follows that economic and demographic changes in the Nation's population are enhancing or mitigating the declining frequency of fluid milk consumption. For example, more Americans are completing college (Cromartie, 2002). The median age of the U.S. population has also increased from 28.1 years in 1970 to 32.9 years in 1990, and 37.2 years in 2010 (Hobbs and Stoops, 2002; Howden and Meyer, 2011).

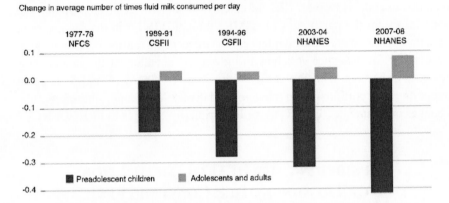

Change in average number of times fluid milk consumed per day

Source: Marginal effects calculated by ERS researchers. Using standard technics for nonlinear models, ERS researchers calculated the marginal effects from data in the 1977-78 Nationwide Food Consumption Survey (NFCS), the 1989-1991 Continuing Survey of Food Intakes by individuals (CSFII), the 1994-1996 CSFII, the 2003-04 National Health and Nutrition Examination Survey (NHANES), and the 2007-08 NHANES.

Notes: Estimates model for FREQUENCY used to calculate marginal effects. In the first step, ERS researchers evaluated the model setting TIME2 through TIME5 equal to zero. In the second step, the researchers re-evaluated the model setting only TIME 2 equal to one, then only TIME3 equal to one, and so on. Finally, results from the first and second steps were compated. Marginal effects are the average differences in the expected value of FREQUENCY between the same individualsof they had participated in 1977-78 survey versus each subsequent survey, all else constant, weighted by sample weight. All effects are negative and statistically significant at the 1-percent level for preadolescent children. However, only effects associated with the 2007-08 NHANE are positive and significant at the 1-percent level for adolescents ande adults. Those for the other surveys are not significantly different than zero.

Figure 8. Marginal effects of time period on fluid milk consumption, all ages.

Portions Remaining Largely Stable

Changes in portions over time appear to contribute little to trends in fluid milk consumption. For both preadolescent children and Americans age 13 and older, estimates of the parameters in the model's second equation reveal a positive relationship between FREQUENCY and QUANTITY. Americans who consume fluid milk on more occasions per day tend to consume a larger quantity overall. However, ERS researchers obtained negative, positive, and zero values for the parameters on TIME2 through TIME5 in the same second equation. Thus, there is no evidence of a trend in quantities consumed after accounting for the other variables in the second equation of the model. This result is consistent with the earlier discussions of figures 4 and 5. It again suggests that portions have changed relatively little and, therefore, that changes over time in QUANTITY reflect primarily changes in FREQUENCY.

CONSIDERING THE HEALTH IMPLICATIONS OF TRENDS IN MILK CONSUMPTION

Americans are consuming less fluid milk, on average, because they drink it on fewer occasions per day. In particular, they drink it less often with their midday and nighttime meals. Mitigating the decline are programs supported by dairy farmers, fluid milk processors, and the Federal Government. Kaiser (2010) confirms that promotions sponsored by checkoff programs increase the demand for fluid milk. Gleason and Suitor (2001) similarly identify a positive association between children's participation in the NSLP and their consumption of fluid milk. These programs moderated the decline in U.S. per capita fluid milk consumption between the 1970s and the 2000s. However, because greater decreases in consumption frequency are observed among more recent generations of Americans, it may be difficult to reverse ongoing consumption trends. Indeed, holding all other factors constant, the gradual replacement in the population of older generations by newer generations will exert downward pressure on Americans' average consumption of fluid milk.

Sustained decreases in per capita fluid milk consumption would work against efforts to raise Americans' overall dairy consumption to recommended levels. To date, Americans have merely maintained their total intake of dairy products by consuming more Cheddar cheese and more mozzarella cheese (USDA-ERS, 2013a). However, the Nation's population would be closer to satisfying dairy recommendations in the *Dietary Guidelines for Americans, 2010* if Americans were still drinking as much fluid milk as they did in the 1970s, in addition to the amounts of other dairy products they now consume.[20] Additionally, cheese products can contain as many or more calories than fluid milk. On a per cup-equivalent basis,[21] regular Cheddar cheese (171 calories) has more calories than a glass of whole milk (149 calories). Whole-fat mozzarella (128 calories) has slightly more calories than 2 percent milk (122 calories). Part-skim mozzarella (108 calories) has slightly more calories than 1 percent milk (102 calories) and somewhat more than skim milk (86 calories).

Nutrition and health policy researchers have warned of the potential health implications of declining fluid milk consumption (e.g., Cavadini et al. 2000; Popkin 2010). If fluid milk consumption continues to decline in response to cohort effects, then raising Americans' dairy intakes and improving overall diet quality would require substantially greater increases in the consumption of non-fluid products in skim and low-fat form. Maintaining a focus on children may also be key to mitigating or halting the downward trend in fluid milk consumption, because habit formation implies that childhood food choices can affect longrun behavior.

APPENDIX I: COMPARING CONSUMPTION ACROSS DIFFERENT USDA DIETARY INTAKE SURVEYS

USDA has been surveying individuals about their dietary intake for several decades. A history of these surveys is available online.[22] The 1977-78 Nationwide Food Consumption Survey (NFCS) was USDA's first survey to be administered nationwide, to cover all four seasons of the year, and to record the food and beverage intakes of a large number of individuals. Subsequent surveys include the 1989-1991 Continuing Survey of Food Intakes by Individuals (CSFII) and the 1994-1996 CSFII. In 2002, the dietary recall portion of the CSFII was integrated with the National Health and Nutrition Examination Survey (NHANES), which is administered by the U.S. Department of Health and Human Services (DHHS). USDA and DHHS now release the results of their integrated survey every 2 years. All of these USDA surveys are nationally representative when analyzed using sample weights.

Pooling food consumption surveys collected intermittently over time is complicated by changes in USDA's survey methodology. For example, in the 1977-78 NFCS and the 1989-91 CSFII, USDA interviewed individuals to complete a 1-day dietary recall for the previous day.[23] Participants then self-reported their own intakes over the subsequent two days (a 2-day diary). By contrast, starting with the 1994-96 CSFII, USDA has interviewed individuals twice to obtain two 1-day dietary recalls for nonconsecutive days. The

NHANES continues to collect multiple 1-day dietary recalls as did the 1994-96 CSFII.

USDA has been consistently administering 1-day dietary recalls for more than 30 years, notwithstanding other changes in survey methodology. It is, therefore, possible to study long-run trends in the American diet by pooling data from only that component of different surveys. Enns et al. (1997) used the 1977-78 NFCS and both CSFIIs to study food consumption trends between the late 1970s and the late 1990s. Cavadini et al. (2000) used these same surveys to focus on dietary trends among American adolescents. Both studies used only the day 1 dietary recall collected shortly after the start of each survey. "This method avoids the biasing of intake results that may occur because of the different dietary data collection methods used ..." (Cavadini et al., 2000, p. 18-19).

USDA has also been improving its protocol for dietary recall interviews since the initial surveys. Research conducted after the 1989-91 CSFII confirmed that survey participants were having difficulty recalling all the foods and beverages consumed the previous day. To aid their memory and reduce the potential for underreporting food intakes, USDA developed a "multiple-pass" protocol. Beginning with the 1994-96 CSFII, interviewers first instructed participants to report all foods and beverages consumed the previous day from midnight to midnight. Then, in a second pass, they asked questions about food items that participants may commonly forget (including, for example, milk on cereal). Finally, in a third pass, interviewers asked questions about eating occasions that survey participants commonly forget. For example, they would ask questions like "Did you nibble or sip on anything while preparing a meal or while waiting to eat that you haven't already told me about?" (see, for example, Tippett and Cypel, 1997). After the merger of the CSFII and NHANES surveys, USDA's three-step methodology was extended to five steps. Studies continue to evaluate the accuracy of dietary recall data collected using the latest multiple-pass protocol (e.g., Conway et al., 2004; Moshfegh et al., 2008).

Because of the introduction of USDA's multiple-pass protocol, it is possible that participants in earlier surveys were more likely to underreport fluid milk consumption than participants in later surveys, though the size of any bias remains unknown. However, figures 1 and 2 reveal that estimates of per capita fluid milk consumption reported in ERS loss-adjusted food availability data are similar to estimates of per capita consumption based on the five USDA food consumption surveys for Americans of all ages. For example, both sources report that Americans, on average, consumed about 1 cup of fluid milk per day in 1977-

78 and about 0.7 cups per day in 2007-08. ERS researchers, therefore, expect that any bias in reported consumption of fluid milk due to the evolution of USDA's multiple-pass protocol is small.

In the current study, ERS researchers focused on fluid milk consumption by participants in USDA surveys over 24 hours. As noted in the text, the researchers included both plain and flavored products consumed alone as a beverage, put in cereal, poured in coffee, or used as an ingredient in selected coffee drinks. USDA dietary records report fluid milk consumption in grams. These quantities were converted into fluid ounces (8 fluid ounces = 1 cup). Quantities of milk consumption were converted from weight to volume by using the USDA National Nutrient Database for Standard Reference, Release 25 (USDA, Agricultural Research Service, 2013b). One 8-ounce cup weighs about 244 grams. The final data set includes information on 64,192 individuals excluding people who failed to provide a reliable day 1 dietary recall, did not provide complete household income or demographic information, or were young children and still breast-feeding.

APPENDIX II: MODEL SPECIFICATION AND ESTIMATION

The Poisson and negative binomial regression models are widely used to analyze count data. In this study, ERS researchers investigated the number of times per day that a person consumes fluid milk (FREQUENCY) and tested whether generational change is contributing to long-run trends in that number. ERS researchers also augmented the basic count data model with a second equation that predicts a survey participant's overall intake of fluid milk (QUANTITY). The goal in adding this second equation was to confirm or refute the possibility that changes in portions sizes are also contributing to trends in fluid milk consumption.

The primary dependent variable in our study, FREQUENCY, can only equal zero or a positive integer value. The probability that it equals a particular value, $0,1,2,3,...,\infty$, using the negative binomial regression model, is:

$$f(FREQUENCY|X) = \frac{\Gamma(FREQUENCY + \theta)}{\Gamma(1 + FREQUENCY)\Gamma(\theta)}\left(\frac{\theta}{\theta+\lambda}\right)^{\theta}\left(\frac{\lambda}{\theta+\lambda}\right)^{FREQUENCY}$$

where $\ddot{e} = e^{\hat{a}x}$ is the conditional mean of FREQUENCY, X is a set of explanatory variables, $\hat{a}$ is a vector of parameters, e is the base of the natural logarithm, $\tilde{A}(\cdot)$ is the gamma function, and $1/\grave{e}$ is the overdispersion parameter. As discussed in the text, if there is no overdispersion, then $\grave{e}$ approaches infinity, the conditional mean and variance of FREQUENCY become equal, and the negative binomial and Poisson regression models become identical.

Among survey participants who consumed fluid milk on zero occasions, both FREQUENCY and QUANTITY equal zero. This occurs with probability

$$P(FREQUENCY=0) = \frac{\Gamma(\theta)}{\Gamma(1)\Gamma(\theta)}\left(\frac{\theta}{\theta+\lambda}\right)^{\theta}.$$

For other survey participants, FREQUENCY and QUANTITY are outcomes of the two variables' joint probability distribution:

$$h(FREQUENCY,QUANTITY|X,Z) = g(QUANTITY| Z)\cdot f(FREQUENCY|X)$$

where f(FREQUENCY|X) is above and g(QUANTITY| Z) is the distribution of QUANTITY conditional on Z. We assume that

$$g(QUANTITY| Z) = \frac{1}{\sqrt{2\pi}\sigma}e^{-\frac{1}{2}\left(\frac{QUANTITY-\alpha Z}{\sigma}\right)^{2}}$$

where $\acute{a}$ is a vector of parameters, e is the base of the natural logarithm, and Z is a set of explanatory variables. That is, we assume $g(\cdot)$ is a normal distribution with mean $\acute{a}Z$ and variance $\acute{o}^{2}$. As discussed in the text, we include FREQUENCY among the variables in Z, but use $\breve{e}=e_{\acute{a}}{}^{x}$ for estimation purposes to reduce the potential for endogeneity bias.

Participants in USDA food consumption surveys must belong to one of two regimes. As noted above, if an individual reported consuming no fluid milk, then both FREQUENCY and QUANTITY equal zero. The contribution to the likelihood function of these individuals follows from the probability of this event as shown above:

$$L1(\beta) = \frac{\Gamma(\theta)}{\Gamma(1)\Gamma(\theta)}\left(\frac{\theta}{\theta+\lambda}\right)^{\theta}$$

For survey participants who consumed fluid milk one or more times, the contribution to the likelihood function is

$$L2(\alpha,\beta) = \frac{1}{\sqrt{2\pi}\sigma} e^{-\frac{1}{2}\left(\frac{QUANTITY - \alpha Z}{\sigma}\right)^2} \frac{\Gamma(FREQUENCY + \theta)}{\Gamma(1 + FREQUENCY)\Gamma(\theta)} \left(\frac{\theta}{\theta + \lambda}\right)^{\theta} \left(\frac{\lambda}{\theta + \lambda}\right)^{FREQUENCY}$$

Finally, the weighted likelihood function for the full sample of i=1,...,N individuals is :

$$L(\alpha,\beta) = \prod_{i=1}^{N} L_i^{w_i}$$

where wi is the sample weight for individual i, Li equals L1 if FREQUENCYi = 0, and Li equals L2 if FREQUENCYi > 0. Estimates of model parameters α and β can be obtained by maximizing the weighted log-likelihood,

$$\ln L(\alpha,\beta) = \sum_{i=1}^{N} w_i \ln L_i .$$

REFERENCES

Bowman, S., S. Gortmaker, C. Ebbeling, M. Pereira, and D. Ludwig. 2004. "Effects of Fast-Food Consumption on Energy Intake and Diet Quality Among Children in a National Household Survey," *Pediatrics*, Vol. 113: pp. 112-118.

Cavadini C., A. Siega-Riz, and B. Popkin. 2000. "U.S. adolescent food intake trends from 1965 to 1996," *Archives of Disease in Childhood*, Vol. 83: pp. 18–24.

Conway J., L. Ingwersen, and A. Moshfegh. 2004. "Accuracy of Dietary Recall Using the USDA Five-Step Multiple-Pass Method in Men: An Observational Validation Study," *Journal of the American Dietetic Association*, Vol. 104: pp. 595-603.

Cromartie J. 2002. "Population Growth and Demographic Change, 1980-2020," *FoodReview*, Vol. 25(1): pp. 10-12. Available at http://www.ers. usda.gov/publications/FoodReview/May2002/DBGen.htm.

Davis C., D. Dong, D. Blayney, and A. Owens. 2010. *An Analysis of U.S. Household Dairy Demand*, TB-1928, U.S. Department of Agriculture,

Economic Research Service. Available at http://www.ers.usda.gov/publications/tb1928/tb1928.pdf .

Deaton A. 1997. *The Analysis of Household Surveys: A Microeconometric Approach to Development Policy*. Baltimore: The Johns Hopkins University Press.

Dong D., P. Byrne, A. Saha, and O. Capps. 2000. "Determinants of Food-Away-FromHome (FAFH) Visit Frequency: A Count-Data Approach," *Journal of Restaurant & Foodservice Marketing*, Vol. 4(1): pp. 31-46.

Efron B., and R. Tibshirani. 1998. *An Introduction to the Bootstrap*. New York: Chapman & Hall.

Enns C., J. Goldman, and A. Cook. 1997. "Trends in Food and Nutrient Intakes by Adults: NFCS 1977-78, CSFII 1989-91, and CSFII 1994-95," *Family Economics and Nutrition Review*, Vol. 10(4): pp. 2-15.

Fisher J., D. Mitchell, H. Smiciklas-Wright, and L. Birch. 2001. "Maternal Milk Consumption Predicts the Tradeoff Between Milk and Soft Drinks in Young Girls' Diets," *Journal of Nutrition,* Vol. 131(2): pp. 246-250.

Gleason P., and C. Suitor. 2001. *Children's Diets in the Mid-1990s: Dietary Intake and Its Relationship with School Meal Participation*, Special Nutrition Programs Report No. CN-01-CD1, U.S. Department of Agriculture, Food and Nutrition Service. Available at http://www.fns.usda.gov/ora/menu/published/CNP/FILES/ChilDiet.pdf

Greene W. 1997. *Econometric Analysis*, 3rd ed., New Jersey: Prentice Hall.

He S., S. Fletcher, and A. Rimal. 2004. "Identifying Factors Influencing Beef, Poultry, and Seafood Consumption," *Journal of Food Distribution Research*, Vol. 34(1): pp. 50-55.

Hobbs F., and N. Stoops. 2002. *Demographic Trends in the 20th Century*, Census 2000 Special Reports, Series CENSR-4, U.S. Department of Commerce, Census Bureau. Available at http://www.census.gov/prod/2002pubs/censr-4.pdf

Howden L., and J. Meyer. 2011. *Age and Sex Composition: 2010*, C2010BR-03, U.S. Department of Commerce, Census Bureau. Available at http://www.census. gov/prod/cen2010/briefs/c2010br-03.pdf

Johnson W. 1980. "Vintage Effects in the Earnings of White American Men," *The Review of Economics and Statistics*, Vol. 62(3): pp. 399-407.

Kaiser H. 2010. *Measuring the Impacts of Generic Fluid Milk and Dairy Marketing*, Research Bulletin 2010-01, Cornell University, National Institute for Commodity Promotion & Research Evaluation. Available at http://dyson.cornell.edu/research/researchpdf/rb/2010/Cornell_Dyson_rb1001.pdf.

Kaiser, H., and D. Dong. 2006. *Measuring the Impacts of Generic Fluid Milk and Dairy Marketing*, Research Bulletin 2006-05, Cornell University, National Institute for Commodity Promotion & Research Evaluation. Available at http://commodity. dyson.cornell.edu/nicpre/bulletins/ rb0605/ rb2006_05.pdf

Lee, E., and R. Forthofer. 2006. *Analyzing Complex Survey Data*, 2nd. ed. Thousand Oaks, California: Sage Publications.

Lin B-H, J. Variyam, J. Allshouse, and J. Cromartie. 2003. *Food and Agricultural Commodity Consumption in the United States: Looking Ahead to 2020*, AER-820, U.S. Department of Agriculture, Economic Research Service. Available at http:// www.ers.usda.gov /Publications/ AER820/ .

Mannino M., Y. Lee, D. Mitchell, H. Smiciklas-Wright, and L. Birch. 2004. "The Quality of Girls' Diets Declines and Tracks Across Middle Childhood," *International Journal of Behavioral Nutrition and Physical Activity,* Vol. 1(5).

Mori H., D. Clason, and J. Lillywhite. 2006. "Estimating Price and Income Elasticities in the Presence of Age-Cohort Effects," *Agribusiness: An International Journal*, Vol. 22(2): pp. 201-217.

Mori H., and Y. Saegusa. 2010. "Cohort Effects in Food Consumption: What They Are and How They Are Formed," *Evolutionary and Institutional Economics Review*, Vol. 7(1): pp. 43–63.

Mori, H., and H. Stewart. 2011. "Cohort Analysis: Ability to Predict Future Consumption – The Cases of Fresh Fruit in Japan and Rice in Korea," *The Annual Bulletin of Social Science*, Vol. 45: pp. 153-173.

Moshfegh A., D. Rhodes, D. Baer, T. Murayi, J. Clemens, W. Rumpler, D. Paul, R. Sebastian, K. Kuczynski, L. Ingwersen, R. Staples, and L. Cleveland. 2008. "The US Department of Agriculture Automated Multiple-Pass Method Reduces Bias in the Collection of Energy Intakes," *American Journal of Clinical Nutrition*, Vol. 88: pp. 324-32.

National Dairy Promotion and Research Board. 2013. Dairy Checkoff Programs. Available at http://www.dairycheckoff.com

Popkin, B. 2010. "Patterns of Beverage Use Across the Lifecycle," *Physiology & Behavior* Vol. 100(1): pp. 4-9.

Schrimper, R. 1979. "Demographic Changes and the Demand for Food: Discussion," *American Journal of Agricultural Economics* 61(5): pp. 1058-60.

Sebastian, R., J. Goldman, C. Enns, and R. LaComb. 2010. "Fluid Milk Consumption in the United States: What We Eat In America, NHANES

2005-2006." 2010. Food Surveys Research Group Dietary Data Brief. No. 3, U.S. Department of Agriculture, Agricultural Research Service. Available at http://ars.usda.gov/SP2UserFiles/ Place/12355000/pdf/ DBrief/fluid_milk_0506.pdf

Stewart, H., D. Dong, and A. Carlson. 2012. "Is generational change contributing to the decline in fluid milk consumption?" *Journal of Agricultural and Resource Economics* Vol. 37(3): pp. 435-54.

Stewart H., and N. Blisard. 2008. "Are Younger Cohorts Demanding Less Fresh Vegetables?" *Review of Agricultural Economics*, Vol. 30(1): pp. 43-60.

Tippett K., and Y. Cypel. 1997. *Design and Operation: The Continuing Survey of Food Intakes by Individuals and the Diet and Health Knowledge Survey, 1994–96*, NFS Report No. 96-1, U.S. Department of Agriculture, Agricultural Research Service. Available at http://www.ars.usda.gov/sp2 userfiles/place/12355000/pdf/Dor9496.pdf.

U.S. Department of Agriculture, Agricultural Research Service. 2013a. *Food and Nutrient Database for Dietary Studies*. Available at http://www. ars.usda.gov/ Services/docs.htm?docid=12089

U.S. Department of Agriculture, Agricultural Research Service. 2013b. *National Nutrient Database for Standard Reference* (Release 25). Available at http:// www.ars.usda.gov/.

U.S. Department of Agriculture, Agricultural Research Service. 2013c. USDA Food Surveys, 1935-1998. Available at http://www.ars.usda.gov/ Services/docs. htm?docid=14392.

U.S. Department of Agriculture, Agricultural Research Service. 2013d. What We Eat in America. Available at http://www.ars.usda.gov/Services/ docs.htm?docid=13793.

U.S. Department of Agriculture, Economic Research Service. 2013a. Loss-Adjusted Food Availability. Available at http://www.ers.usda.gov/Data/ FoodCon sumption/FoodGuideIndex.htm/.

U.S. Department of Agriculture, Economic Research Service. 2013b. Food Availability (Per Capita) Data System. Available at http://www. ers.usda.gov/Data/ FoodConsumption/

U.S. Department of Agriculture and U.S. Department of Health and Human Services. 2010. *Dietary Guidelines for Americans, 2010* 7th ed. Washington, DC, December. Available at http://www.cnpp.usda.gov/ dietaryguidelines.htm

End Notes

[1] Popkin (2010) examined the consumption of milks, sugar-sweetened beverages (SSB), diet beverages, juices, alcoholic beverages, and unsweetened tea and coffee. SSBs include carbonated and uncarbonated soft drinks, sugared waters, and energy drinks, among others. He studied consumption trends for children and adolescents aged 2 to 18 years. Popkin (2010) separately examined beverage consumption for adults aged 19 and older.

[2] The Dietary Guidelines for Americans, 2010 are issued by USDA and the U.S. Department of Health and Human Services (DHHS) to provide evidence-based nutrition information and advice for people age 2 and older. They also serve as the nutritional basis for Federal food and nutrition assistance education programs.

[3] A checkoff program collects funds from producers of a particular agricultural commodity and uses these funds to promote and conduct research on that commodity.

[4] These data are created by adjusting food availability data for food spoilage and other forms of food loss to better proxy for consumption. Loss-adjusted food availability data are not available prior to 1970.

[5] Whole milk has a minimum fat content of 3.25 percent. ERS researchers were not able to separately identify consumption trends for 2 percent (reduced-fat), 1 percent (low-fat), and skim milk. As noted in the text above, current dietary recommendations place special emphasis on low-fat and skim milk.

[6] Recipes developed for use with more recent food consumption surveys are available in the USDA Food and Nutrient Database for Dietary Studies (FNDDS). See USDA, Agricultural Research Service (2013a).

[7] Includes only coffee drinks that are 50 percent or more milk such as a latte (75 percent milk), café con leche (51 percent), mocha (66 percent), cappuccino (51 percent), and sweetened milk coffee with ice (58 percent).

[8] Americans consume only a small amount of soy beverages compared with their consumption of cow's milk. ERS researchers confirmed that including the former in the analysis would not significantly affect the study's results.

[9] Midday meal is defined as a meal occasion occurring between 11 a.m. and 5 p.m.

[10] Individuals born prior to 1930 would not have likely been influenced as preadolescent children by the changes in milk consumption that started in the 1940s. ERS researchers, therefore, hypothesized that generational effects exist only for Americans born in 1930 or more recently.

[11] For example, given that the other explanatory variables included a person's income, demographic characteristics, and his or her birth year, ERS researchers could interpret the results on TIME5 to answer the question, "If the same population that existed in 1977-78 still existed in 2007-08, how much would consumption have fallen or risen?"

[12] The Bureau of Labor Statistics (BLS) has been publishing a CPI for whole fresh milk since at least the 1970s and a CPI for fresh milk other than whole milk since 1997. The two series have moved together closely. Changes in the two CPIs share a correlation coefficient of 0.98 in the years for which both indices are available.

[13] Unobservable differences in tastes, dietary knowledge, and medical conditions between individuals could contribute to the error terms in both our equations for FREQUENCY and QUANTITY. That is, these omitted variables could affect both the frequency of consumption and portion sizes. This would then lead to endogeneity bias.

[14] This is an instrumental variable approach.

[15] Sample weights provided by USDA for use with its surveys were incorporated into the estimation.

[16] Consistent with test results for adolescents and adults, ERS researchers noted that the mean of FREQUENCY (0.81) was less than the variance of FREQUENCY (1.01). This was not the case for preadolescent children. FREQUENCY had a mean and variance of 1.65 and 1.43 among survey respondents in this age group, respectively.

[17] Efron and Tibshirani (1998, p. 52) report that 100 replications "gives quite satisfactory results" and "very seldom" are more than 200 replications needed. For this study, ERS researchers used 250 replications. Each replication included 64,192 observations drawn from the original sample with replacement and a probability proportional to the sample weight (Efron and Tibshirani, 1998; Lee and Forthofer, 2006).

[18] For example, ERS checked that the findings on C2 through C14 for adolescents and adults were not driven by any correlation with changes in prices, changes in the availabilities of milk and competing beverages, or changes in other factors correlated with time. This was accomplished by re-estimating the equation for FREQUENCY for adolescents and adults excluding all time variables, TIME2 through TIME5. Estimation results on C2 through C14 were qualitatively unchanged, confirming the robustness of our findings.

[19] ERS estimated these effects for each individual in the sample. They then used the sample weights to calculate the weighted averaged effect across all individuals. See also notes to figures 7 and 8.

[20] ERS food availability data show that Americans consume 1.53 cup-equivalents of dairy products, on average, including 0.61 cup-equivalents of fluid milk (USDA-ERS, 2013a). Thus, raising fluid milk consumption to 0.96 cup-equivalents per person, as in the early 1970s, would raise the per capita total to about 2 cup-equivalents. As noted above, The Dietary Guidelines for Americans, 2010 recommends 2 cup-equivalents per day for children aged 2 to 3 years, 2.5 for those aged 4 to 8 years, and 3 for Americans older than age 8.

[21] Consuming 8 ounces of fluid milk, 1.5 ounces of Cheddar cheese, or 1.5 ounces of mozzarella cheese all count equally toward an individual's consumption of dairy products. Each is considered to be 1 cup-equivalent. Each is also available in higher and lower fat forms. ERS researchers used the USDA National Nutrient Database for Standard Reference, Release 25 (USDA, Agricultural Research Service, 2013b) to compare the number of calories in selected forms of these foods' per cup-equivalents.

[22] See USDA, Agricultural Research Service (2013c, 2013d).

[23] In the 1977-78 NFCS, USDA also collected information on household food use over a 1-week period. In the 1989-91 CSFII, USDA ceased to collect household food use data and concentrated exclusively on the diets of individuals.

In: Milk Consumption
Editor: Francisco Paul Buren

Chapter 2

HOUSEHOLDS' CHOICES AMONG FLUID MILK PRODUCTS: WHAT HAPPENS WHEN INCOME AND PRICES CHANGE?*

Diansheng Dong and Hayden Stewart

ABSTRACT

Households have several ways to economize on their purchases at retail food stores when prices increase or their incomes fall. This report investigates a household's choice among retail fluid milk products categorized along three dimensions: three levels of fat content, two levels of package size, and organic versus conventional methods of production. Nielsen Homescan data from 2007-08 are used to estimate a choice model, which accounts for price, income, and other choice determinants. Results show that small changes in prices and income have a modest impact on a household's choice among milk products. However, households mitigate the impact of more substantial price and income shocks by switching from more expensive to less expensive products. We also find that the demand for organic milk is more sensitive to swings in income and food prices than is demand for conventional milk.

---

* This is an edited, reformatted and augmented version of theUnited States Department of Agriculture publication, Economic Research Report Number 146 dated April 2013.

Keywords: Milk purchases, milk prices, dairy product, dairy prices, organic milk, household income, household food economizing behavior, Homescan data, fluid milk, recession

SUMMARY

What Is the Issue?

Many households experienced a decrease in income during the 2007-2009 recession. At the same time, food prices rose. In 2008, the median U.S. household made 3.6 percent less money after adjustment for inflation than it did in 2007, while prices for fluid milk at retail food stores rose 11.6 percent in 2007 and 6 percent in 2008. Households have several ways to economize on their retail food purchases when prices increase or their incomes fall. More information on how households economize on their purchases may help policymakers better understand the relationship of consumer choices to changes in the economy and to a host of demographic variables.

What Did the Study Find?

Households experiencing an income decrease may look for ways to stretch their food dollar, such as seeking out promotions or shopping at less expensive stores like supercenters. This study focuses on the type of fluid milk a household buys. Fluid milk that is higher fat, organic, or packaged in small containers is more expensive per gallon than milk that is lower fat, conventionally produced, or packaged in large containers. Households typically switch to less expensive products when their incomes decrease. For instance, households save money by choosing fluid milk products with a lower fat content or by switching from organic to conventional milk.

Households with an increase in income, however, do not always buy more expensive products:

A 10-percent increase in household income:

- Raises the probability of purchasing organic milk from 3 to 3.7 percent;

- Raises the probability of buying low-fat milk (defined as "skim and less than 2 percent fat") from 47 to 48.6 percent;
- Lowers the probability of purchasing whole milk (at least 3.25 percent fat) from 17 to 15.9 percent;
- Lowers the probability of choosing reduced-fat milk (between 2 and 3.25 percent fat) from 36 to 35.5 percent; and
- Has only a small effect on households' choice among products in different container sizes.

Changes in retail prices also affect a household's choice among different milk products:

- A small (1-percent) increase in prices for all milk products has only a small effect on the division of sales among products with different levels of fat content and in different package sizes, as well as division of sales between milk produced using conventional and organic methods.
- A large ($1 per gallon or approximately 25-percent) increase in retail milk prices is large enough to curb growth in sales of organic milk.
- A large increase in prices for all milk products also increases the probability— from 47 to 53.9 percent—of purchasing low-fat milk.
- Even large price shocks have little effect on households' choice between package sizes. The probability of purchasing milk in a container smaller than 1 gallon decreases from 42 to 40.2 percent.

Overall, when substantial price and income shocks occur, households switch from more expensive to less expensive products. This practice may help households afford a healthful diet when budgets get tight. However, many lower income Americans already (before income reductions or general price increases) purchase less expensive items; likewise, lower income households are less likely to choose organic milk. This lack of flexibility may render households already on a tight budget more exposed to the effects of price volatility.

In general, demand for organic milk is more sensitive than demand for conventional milk to swings in income and food prices. Past research suggests that many buyers of organic milk question conventional production methods and believe organic products to be safer and/or more healthful. Nonetheless, during the recent recession, when incomes declined and prices rose, growth in organic milk sales stalled.

How Was the Study Conducted?

We investigate a household's choice among retail fluid milk products categorized along three dimensions: three levels of fat content, two levels of package size, and organic versus conventional methods of production. Categorizing retail products along all 3 dimensions yields 12 specific products (e.g., low-fat organic milk in a 1-gallon container). A unique multinomial logit choice model is applied to account for past household purchase behavior, price, promotional deal, and seasonality. It also accounts for household demographic variables such as income and number of household members, as well as the age, employment status, education, and ethnicity of the head of household and whether or not the home was owned. We use 2007- 2008 Nielsen Homescan data to estimate the choice model. Finally, using model results for each of the 12 specific products, we simulate how shocks to prices, income, and other demand determinants would affect the probability that a household buys lower fat versus higher fat fluid milk, conventional or organic products, and fluid milk packaged in a 1-gallon or smaller container.

INTRODUCTION

Households may need to stretch their food dollars either when their incomes decrease or when food prices increase. Many Americans experienced both of these conditions during the December 2007 to June 2009 recession. This report examines the question of how consumers adjust their choices when faced with income and price shocks for a staple (in this report, fluid milk), which is available in a variety of retail forms and container sizes.

Households have several ways to economize on their purchases at retail food stores when prices increase or their incomes fall. They may buy smaller quantities of some foods, but ultimately, they need to eat. Aside from buying less food, Leibtag and Kaufman (2003), for example, show that households may adjust their purchase behavior by shopping at less expensive stores or substituting less expensive foods. This project focuses on the second possibility: we investigate households' choices among fluid milk products (1) sold in gallon versus less-than-gallon containers, (2) produced using organic versus conventional methods, and (3) containing more and less milk fat. That is, when prices and income change along with other variables, how do households adjust their choices among these substitute fluid milk products?

The median U.S. household saw its income fall 3.6 percent in 2008 and 0.7 percent in 2009 after adjustment for inflation.[1] In addition, food prices had already begun to rise in early 2007. Food price inflation reached 4 percent in 2007 and 5.5 percent in 2008 before moderating to 1.8 percent in 2009.[2] Foods that became substantially more expensive included staples like fluid milk. Prices for milk at retail food stores rose 11.6 percent in 2007 and 6 percent in 2008 before ultimately falling 13.2 percent in 2009.[3]

The price of 2 percent milk rose above $4 per gallon in many U.S. cities during the 2007-08 peak of inflation.[4] Kumcu and Kaufman (2011) show that, in general, consumers reacted to the combination of lower incomes and higher food prices over these years by economizing on their food purchases. They took advantage of sales, promotions, and coupons; substituted comparable, but lower cost foods; and sought stores with lower prices and more cost-effective selections.

Fluid milk is a staple of the American diet, and it is especially important to young people. Americans consumed about 0.75 cup per day, on average, in 2005-06 (Sebastian et al., 2010), and during those same years, children ages 2 to 11 consumed between 1.25 and 1.5 cups per day. Cornick et al. (1994) found that 96.1 percent of all households bought fluid milk over a 1-year period in the early 1990s.

Furthermore, the *Dietary Guidelines for Americans, 2010* encourages consumption of dairy products.[5] Americans are advised that consuming enough dairy products can improve bone health and lower blood pressure, as well as reduce the risk of cardiovascular disease and type 2 diabetes. However, "most" Americans aged 4 and over consume less than the recommended quantity of dairy products (p. 38).

Although milk has long been considered a major food product to provide necessary nutrients such as calcium, milk fat has also been viewed as a contributor to obesity in America. Fat-free and low-fat fluid milk provide necessary nutrients, such as calcium, with fewer calories than higher fat dairy products. Thus, the type of milk a household buys plays a role in its members' health. Whether or not consumers substitute between whole milk and lower fat products will affect not only their budgets, but also how closely they adhere to Federal dietary guidelines.

In addition to affecting health, consumer choices of milk products influence dairy production trends. One example of such influence is in organic dairy production. Organic dairy farmers represent a small but growing share of the overall market for fluid milk. To qualify for certification under USDA's National Organic Program, conventional milk producers must undergo a process that can be challenging and costly (McBride and Greene, 2009). To help cover those costs and support the recent growth in organic dairy farming, farmers have largely relied on the willingness of many consumers to pay a premium for organic milk. Smith et al. (2009), for example, find that the organic premium for a half-gallon of low-fat milk is between 72 and 88 percent, depending on whether the milk is also branded. Because of the financial risk involved, conventional milk producers thinking of switching to organic production need information not only on consumers' willingness to pay, but on the robustness of that willingness, in the face of price and income shocks.

In this report, we investigate a household's choice among retail fluid milk products categorized along three dimensions: three levels of fat content,[6] two levels of package size ("1 gallon" and "less-than-gallon sized"), and organic versus conventional methods of production. Categorizing retail products along all 3 dimensions (e.g., low-fat organic milk in a 1-gallon container) yields 12 specific products. We estimate a choice model that allows predicting the effects of changes in prices and income, among other factors, on a household's choices among the 12 products. Results obtained in this study may help policymakers better understand the relationship of consumer choices to changes in the economy and to a host of demographic variables.

Households' Purchases of Fluid Milk

When prices rise or incomes fall, consumers tend to reduce the quantity of milk that they consume by a proportionally smaller amount. A review of existing research by Andreyeva et al. (2010) identifies 26 studies that estimate the price elasticity of demand for milk using either time series or cross-sectional data. The average reported estimate was -0.59, meaning that if the price of milk were to increase (or decrease) by 10 percent, the expected decrease (or increase) in the quantity consumed would be only 6 percent. However, during the past recession, despite the rise of milk prices and fall of incomes, quantities of milk consumed were unusually stable. Loss-adjusted food availability data reveal that per capita consumption remained about 14.5 gallons per person per year (USDA-ERS, 2012).

In a recession or when prices increase, households may seek to economize in ways other than consuming less of staple foods. One way is shopping at less expensive stores. Dong and Stewart (2012) show that, after an income decrease, a household is more likely to buy fluid milk at a supercenter than at either a traditional grocery store or club warehouse. Another way that households may economize is by substituting less expensive products for more expensive ones.

For the analysis, we use 2007 and 2008 Nielsen Homescan data to investigate a household's choices among retail milk products. Nielsen maintains a consumer panel that demographically and geographically represents the continental United States. Participating households from all 48 contiguous States are given scanners to keep in their homes. After a shopping occasion, panelists use these scanners to record food purchases, including the Universal Product Code (UPC), the quantities bought, the amount of money paid, the purchase date, and price promotions, if any. The data are likewise daily transaction data and include purchases at all grocery retail stores. Homescan panelists do not record purchases at foodservice outlets including restaurants and, most importantly, in the case of fluid milk, schools.

It is possible that some households make mistakes when reporting information to Nielsen (e.g., some may fail to report all purchases because the recording process is time consuming). However, Einav et al. (2008) analyze the accuracy of these data and find that errors in Homescan data are of the same order of magnitude as reporting errors in Government-collected data sets commonly used to measure earnings and employment status.

The Homescan data used in this study include information on purchases by 24,110 households. For each of these, Nielsen provides detailed information on each transaction as well as information on each household's demographic characteristics and county of residence.

The data confirm that most American households buy fluid milk. Although prices rose in 2007, the Homescan data show that 95.2 percent of households still bought fluid milk that year, about 0.9 percent less than reported by Cornick et al. (1994). In 2008, 94.8 percent of households bought fluid milk.

Retail food stores typically offer a wide array of fluid milk products. We divide this array along three dimensions (table 1). The first of these dimensions is fat content, with levels defined as *whole* (at least 3.25 percent fat), *reduced-fat* (between 2 and 3.25 percent milk fat), and *low fat* (less than 2 percent milk fat). Other product dimensions include package size (i.e., gallon or in smaller sized packages), and, finally, whether milk is produced by conventional or organic methods.

Table 1. Fluid milk products and marketing variables

Fluid milk product descriptions (by fat content, container size, and means of production)	Average daily price	Average daily share of sales made on a deal	Purchase frequency annual and seasonal				
			Annual	Winter	Spring	Summer	Fall
	Dollars per gallon	Percent			Percent		
1 Whole, 1 gallon, conventional	3.57	14.6	8.8	8.8	8.9	8.7	9.1
2 Reduced-fat, 1 gallon, conventional	3.38	17.5	20.8	20.7	20.6	20.7	21.1
3 Low-fat, 1 gallon, conventional	3.27	19.7	27.5	27.5	27.5	27.6	27.4
4 Whole, less than gallon, conventional	5.30	9.9	7.8	8.0	7.6	7.8	7.9
5 Reduced-fat, less than gallon, conventional	5.04	13.3	14.0	13.9	14.0	14.1	13.8
6 Low-fat, less than gallon, conventional	4.93	15.3	18.1	18.1	18.4	18.1	17.6
7 Whole, 1 gallon, organic	5.60	20.2	0.1	0.1	0.1	0.1	0.1
8 Reduced-fat, big 1 gallon, organic	5.24	11.7	0.1	0.1	0.1	0.1	0.2
9 Low-fat, 1 gallon, organic	5.21	18.8	0.3	0.3	0.3	0.3	0.4
10 Whole, less than gallon, organic	7.28	19.0	0.5	0.5	0.5	0.5	0.4
11 Reduced-fat, less than gallon, organic	7.19	17.7	0.7	0.7	0.7	0.7	0.7
12 Low-fat, less than gallon, organic	7.15	21.3	1.3	1.4	1.3	1.4	1.2

Source: Calculated by authors using 2007-08 Nielsen Homescan data.

Note: Average daily prices for each of the 12 products are the average prices over all the dates of the year. Other values in the table are proportions. Gallon-sized containers of conventional low-fat or skim milk accounted for 27.5 percent of all purchases annually and were the most often purchased product.

Low-fat milk is defined as less than 2 percent fat including skim; reduced-fat is between 2 and 3.25 percent fat; and whole is at least 3.25 percent fat.

Dividing retail milk products along all 3 dimensions produces 12 distinct milk products. For example, conventionally produced, low-fat milk in a gallon container is the most frequently bought product (28 percent of all purchases), while organic whole and organic reduced-fat milk sold in gallon containers tie for least frequently bought (both with less than 0.1 percent of total sales). The prices used in this report are average daily prices paid by households for each of the 12 different milk products.[7] Over 2007-08, the least expensive product was conventional low-fat milk sold by the gallon for $3.27 (table 1). The most expensive was organic whole milk sold in a less-than-gallon container at $7.28 per gallon.

Products may have also been purchased while being promoted by either a manufacturer or a store. Promotional deals include manufacturer coupons, store coupons, and store features, among others. The promotional deal variable is the share of each day's purchases of each product that were made on promotion.

What are the most purchased types of milk products? When the 2007-2008 retail market is sorted according to products' fat content, low-fat and skim milk accounted for 47 percent of all purchases by U.S households; reduced-fat milk accounted for 36 percent; and whole milk accounted for 17 percent of all purchases. Regarding container size and organic purchases, the research shows that households bought milk in a gallon-sized container 58 percent of the time, and all six organic products collectively accounted for about 3 percent of all purchases.

Casual observation reveals that food retailers often sell whole, reduced-fat, and low-fat milk for the same price, but, on average, they sell higher fat products at a higher price. Consider prices paid for conventional milk packaged in a less-thangallon container. Consumers paid $4.93 per gallon for low-fat milk versus $5.30 for similarly packaged, conventionally produced, whole milk (table 1)—a premium of $0.37 per gallon. Under Federal milk marketing orders, the minimum price paid to farmers for fluid milk is higher for higher fat products. Fat extracted from fluid milk is valuable because it is used to make other dairy products like cream and butter.

Cornick et al. (1994) and, more recently, Davis et al. (2010) examine the effects of a household's income and demographic characteristics on its purchases of whole and lower fat milk products. Davis et al. (2010) find that Black households and households with young children purchase more whole milk than other households. By contrast, high-income households and households whose female head of household has attended college tend to buy more lower fat products.

Another of this report's product dimensions considers the variety of fluid-milk package sizes, the most common being the gallon container. Buying milk this way costs less per gallon. Consumers paid $3.27 for conventional low-fat milk in a gallon container versus $4.93 per gallon for this same type of milk in smaller containers—a premium of $1.66 per gallon (table 1). Though it stands to reason that lower income households might economize by purchasing products in larger containers, Leibtag and Kaufman (2003) find that lower income households are less likely to take advantage of economy-sized packages for ready-to-eat cereal, meat, poultry, fruits, vegetables, and cheese, among other products. One possible explanation is that households living on a tight budget cannot afford to "stock up" on staples. Another is that lower income households have less storage space in their homes. The data used by Leibtag and Kaufman (2003) did not include fluid milk.

The study's third product dimension tracks whether fluid milk purchases were produced using organic or conventional methods. McBride and Greene (2009) note that conventional dairy farmers switching to organic production must make changes in animal husbandry, alter land and crop management, and secure organic feed, among other endeavors. The process can be challenging and costly. Sales of organic milk have, nonetheless, grown rapidly since the 1990s.

Chronicling this growth, Dupuis (2000) notes that many buyers of organic milk question conventional production methods and believe organic products to be safer and/or more healthful. The use of the hormone Recombinant Bovine Somatotropin (rBST) to increase production yields was once particularly controversial. Several studies have since measured the premium that some consumers are willing to pay for organic milk. As noted above, Smith et al. (2009) demonstrate that this premium can be substantial. Kiesel and Villas-Boas (2007) find that the USDA organic seal increases the probability of purchasing organic milk.

Despite these findings, growth in organic milk sales stalled during the recent recession. Organic products accounted for 2.7 percent of all U.S.-marketed fluid milk in December 2007 at the onset of the recession.[8] That share was nearly unchanged at 2.8 percent in December 2009, about 6 months after the recession had ended. Growth did eventually recover along with the economy. Organic products accounted for 3.9 percent of all milk marketed in the United States in December 2011.

When prices rise or incomes fall, do buyers of organic milk switch back to conventional products? And what determines which consumers choose to buy organic milk and which continue to choose conventional products? Dhar and Foltz (2005) estimate a demand model for organic milk products, conventional milk labeled as rBST-free, and unlabeled conventional milk. They find that the demand for organic products is more price sensitive than the demand for unlabeled conventional products.

Also, they confirm that unlabeled conventional milk is a substitute for organic milk. A later study by Alviola and Capps (2010) finds that the demand for organic milk is also relatively more sensitive to changes in income. Moreover, the demand for organic milk varies with a person's level of education, race, ethnicity, and household size, among other things. College-educated households in particular are more likely to exhibit a preference for organic milk over conventional products.

Milk Purchase Choice Model

Our review of existing research on the demand for milk by American households reveals that households make purchase choices based partly on the attributes of the available products and partly on prices and the use of promotional deals. For example, Dhar and Foltz (2005) find that the demand for organic products is price sensitive, although other studies like Smith et al. (2009) also show that some households are willing to pay a significant premium. These households may feel that organic products are safer and/or more healthful.

Also important are a household's own characteristics, which can cause it to exhibit a preference for a particular type of milk product. These characteristics include not only income and demographics, as discussed above, but also past purchase history.

Guadagni and Little (1983) demonstrate that habit formation can significantly affect food choices. Specifically, in a study of a household's choice among various ground coffee products, Guadagni and Little (1983) demonstrate that a household may choose a particular type of product and thereafter exhibit a tendency to choose that same product in the future. Among the demographic characteristics of households, it has been demonstrated that income, level of educational attainment, household size, race, and ethnicity, among other factors, can influence the type of milk a household consumes (e.g., Davis et al., 2010).

We now estimate a choice model that accounts for the major determinants of a household's choice among fluid milk products. The multinomial logit model has been widely used to study a household's choice among food products in general.

However, the standard form of this model does not account for all of the key choice determinants. To obtain a satisfactory model, we instead start by defining a consumer's utility over the 12 milk products analyzed in this report. For household i, the utility to buy food product j at time t is defined as follows:

$$U_{ijt} = \alpha_j + \beta X_{jt} + L_{ijt}(\theta; Y_{ijt-1}, Z_i) + \varepsilon_{ijt} \tag{1}$$

where α_j is an intercept that captures the contribution to consumer utility of the attributes associated with food product j. X_{jt} is a vector of marketing variables, such as prices and any promotional deals for product j at time t. X_{jt} may also account for the season of the year. β and θ are vectors of parameters to be estimated. L_{ijt} is a household characteristic variable whose value is determined by the household's demographic characteristics (Z_i) and past purchasing history y_{ijt-1} prior to time t. $Yijt-1$ can be defined as a $(t-1) \times 1$ vector of 0's and 1's with the rth element equal to 1 if household i purchased product j at time r and equal to zero otherwise. In research on choice models, L_{ijt} is commonly called the "loyalty variable," because it accounts for a household's past purchase history, among other things. Finally, as in Guadagni and Little (1983), we assume that household utility further contains a random component, ε_{ijt}.

Alternative approaches for modeling a household's choice among competing food products include the random coefficient logit model. This model allows for household heterogeneity by assuming that β is randomly distributed across households. However, the estimation of a random coefficient model usually requires the evaluation of high order probability integrals. Therefore, the model in (1) is relatively much easier to estimate. Also, we can use L_{ijt} to differentiate utility U_{ijt} among households. We can, therefore, explicitly model the effects of household demographic variables and a household's past purchase history, as discussed further below—something not possible using a traditional random coefficient logit model.

The specification of the loyalty variable, $_{Lijt,}$ to incorporate household characteristics into choice models is a subject of much research. Guadagni and Little (1983) propose a specification that uses a weighted average of past choice behavior. Recent choices are weighted more heavily. Fader and Lattin (1993) propose an alternative specification in which habits can change with sudden, unforeseen events. For example, a promotional campaign may cause a consumer to try a new product. However, both studies ignore household demographics. Dong and Stewart (2012) expand on Fader and Lattin's (1993) approach by additionally including household demographics in $_{Lijt.}$ In this study, we follow Dong and Stewart (2012) to account for both household demographics and past purchase behavior in specifying variable $Lijt$ (See appendix I.)

A household chooses among products to maximize utility. The probability that household i selects product j at time t is therefore $p_{ijt} = \text{Prob}(U_{ijt} > U_{ikt})$ for all k not equal to j. If we further assume the random component in utility, ε_{ijt}, is an independently distributed random variable with a type II extreme value (double exponential) distribution, the value of p_{ijt} is

$$p_{ijt} = \frac{e^{U_{ijt}}}{\sum_{l=1}^{J} e^{U_{ilt}}}$$

(2)

which serves as the basis of our multinomial logit choice model.

An assumption of the multinomial logit model is that the odds ratios, p_j/p_k, based on equation (2) are independent of the other alternatives. This assumption is the so-called "Independence from Irrelevant Alternatives" (IIA), and it stipulates that the choice alternatives in the model are mutually independent. If this assumption is violated, systematic errors will occur in the predicted choice probabilities (Guadagni and Little 1983). We use the Hausman-McFadden approach (Hausman and McFadden, 1984) to test the validity of this assumption for the empirical model.

Another assumption of the model is that households choose only one type of milk at a time. For example, if household i bought two types milk at time t, we would treat these purchases as two separate purchase occasions on which one type of milk was bought. Dube (2004) developed a model that can handle multiple purchase units using a Poisson model to predict the number of consumption occasions across all household members. However, similar to the random coefficient logit model, Dube's (2004) model also requires evaluating high order probability integrals. In our data, only 5.25 percent of all purchases were made on the same day as another type of milk was bought.

The log likelihood function for this multinomial logit choice model, given a purchase history $_{(yijt),}$ can be written as

$$\ln L = \sum_{i=1}^{N} \sum_{j=1}^{J} \sum_{t=1}^{T} y_{ijt} \ln p_{ijt}$$

(3)

where N is the total number of households, T is the total number of purchase occasions, and J is the total number of alternative products to be chosen. Model estimates can be obtained from maximizing equation (3).

The marginal effect of X, the seasonality and marketing variables, on the product choice probabilities can be derived from equation (2) for household i as

$$\frac{\partial P_{ij}}{\partial X_l} = \begin{cases} P_{ij}(1-P_{ij})\beta, & if \ l = j \\[2ex] -P_{ij}P_{il}\beta, & if \ l \neq j \end{cases} \tag{4}$$

where P_{ij} is the average probability of household i purchasing product j over all the purchase occasions. The associated elasticity can be written as:

$$\frac{\partial P_{ij}}{\partial X_l}\frac{X_l}{P_{ij}} = X_l(1-P_{ij}) \cdot \beta \ \text{for} \ l = j \ \text{and} \ \ \frac{\partial P_{ij}}{\partial X_l}\frac{X_l}{P_{ij}} = -X_l P_{ij} \cdot \beta \ \text{for} \ l \neq j.$$

where X_l is the vector of average seasonality and marketing variables associated with product l over all the purchase occasions.

The household variables Z_i are incorporated into the household loyalty variable L_{ijt}. The elasticity of product choice probability with respect to Z_i can be derived from equation (2) as

$$\eta_{jz} = \frac{\partial P_{ij}}{\partial Z_i}\frac{Z_i}{P_{ij}} = (\frac{1}{L_{ij}}\frac{\partial L_{ij}}{\partial Z_i} - \sum_{l=1}^{J} P_{il}\frac{1}{L_{il}}\frac{\partial L_{il}}{\partial Z_i}) \cdot Z_i \tag{5}$$

where all the variables are the average values over all the purchase occasions by household i.

We use the Homescan data described above to create all the variables needed in both X and Z. The marketing variables (X) used in this study include milk price, promotional deal, and seasonal dummies (table 1). Based on previous milk purchase studies, we include the following among demographic variables: household income, household size, age, employment, education level of the female household head, and household ethnicity in Z. The presence of small children and teenagers usually influences household milk consumption, so we further include binary variables to indicate if households have small children (younger than 6) and young teenagers (between 13 and 17). We also include a dummy variable to indicate single-person households, because single people may behave differently from other types of households regarding food purchases. To capture variation in milk demand across households living in rural/suburban communities and inner-city neighborhoods, we include a population density variable (the population per square mile in a household's county of residence). Summary statistics for the demographic variables are provided in table 2.

Table 2. Household variables

Variable	Mean	Std. Err	Min	Max
Household income (in dollars)	60,164	40,317	2,500	250,000
Household size (number of people)	2.23	1.17	1	9
Age of female head (in years)	55.99	10.31	22	68
Population density of the household residential area	1,547	5,056	0.76	70,924
Employment: = 1 if female head employed; = 0 if not	0.41	0.49	0	1
Education: = 1 if female head gained college education; = 0 if not	0.38	0.49	0	1
House: = 1 if owned house; = 0 if not	0.81	0.39	0	1
Single: = 1 if household size is 1; = 0 if not	0.27	0.44	0	1
Black: = 1 if household is African American; = 0 if other	0.08	0.28	0	1
Hisp: = 1 if household is Hispanic; = 0 if not	0.05	0.22	0	1
AgeC6: = 1 if presence of children 6 and below; = 0 if not	0.04	0.19	0	1
AgeC1317: = 1 if presence of children between 13 and 17; = 0 if not	0.10	0.29	0	1

Source: Calculated by authors using 2007-08 Nielsen Homescan data.

The household income was converted to a continuous variable from 33 discrete categories using the mean of each category. For the highest category, $250K and above, we use $250K. Similarly, the age variable is converted to a continuous variable from the 29 discrete categories provided in the data.

Many Underlying Factors to Households' Product Choices

The multinomial logit model in equation (2) was estimated using the data on 24,110 Homescan households over 730 days (the 2 years of 2007 and 2008). Each household could have bought milk on each of these days. Households made an average of 58 purchases during the 2 years. The total number of milk purchases (observations) in the data is 1,390,263. The log likelihood in equation (3) was maximized using GAUSS software. The standard errors of the estimated parameters were then obtained from the inverse of the numerically evaluated Hessian matrix of the likelihood function (parameter estimates, standard errors, and the value of the log likelihood function evaluated at these parameter estimates are reported in the appendix II).

As mentioned above, the multinomial logit choice model assumes IIA. To test this assumption, we follow Hausman and McFadden (1984). We re-ran the model including only the six conventional milk products and dropping all six of the organic milk products. Suppose γ_0 is the vector of all the parameter estimates for the subset model with the variance-covariance matrix Ω_0, and γ_1 is the vector of the associated parameter estimates with γ_0 for the full model with the variance-covariance matrix Ω_1. Then,

$$\chi^2(r) = (\gamma_1 - \gamma_0)'(\Omega_1 - \Omega_0)^{-1}(\gamma_1 - \gamma_0) \tag{6}$$

has a chi-square distribution with the degrees of freedom r when IIA is true, where r is the rank of $\Omega_1 - \Omega_0$. In our test, $\alpha^2 = 96.8$ with 89 degrees of freedom. The 5-percent critical value for the test is 112, which implies that we cannot reject IIA at the 0.05 significance level.

For each of the 12 milk products, we then used the estimation results to calculate how much the probability of choosing each product would change with prices, promotional deals, income, household size, age, and other variables. Specifically, we calculated the elasticities of the choice probabilities. For the continuous explanatory variables, the elasticities are evaluated at the means of the explanatory variables and are best interpreted as the percentage changes in the probability of buying a particular milk product with a 1-percent change in the choice determinant. For the discrete explanatory variables, the elasticities are the percentage changes in the probability of buying a particular milk product when the discrete variable changes from 0 to 1. The standard errors of all elasticities were calculated from the Delta method proposed by Rao (1973). The results are reported in tables 3 to 5.

Income and Demographics

Households are hypothesized to switch from higher to lower priced milk products when their food budgets get tight. However, when incomes change, it is primarily the demand for organic milk products that is affected. Higher income households will purchase more organic milk (table 3). The largest increase in purchase probability is for low-fat, organic milk in a small container. On the one hand, buying less expensive products may help households with reduced incomes to afford a healthful diet.

Table 3. Percentage changes in probability of purchasing fluid milk with respect to a 1-percent change in household variables

	Percentage changes in purchase probability						
	WHBC	RFBC	LFBC	WHSC	RFSC	LFSC	WHBO
HH ncome	-0.2315*	-0.1005*	0.0588*	-0.0941*	-0.0155*	0.1063*	0.0410
	(0.0063)	(0.0039)	(0.0046)	(0.0060)	(0.0042)	(0.0038)	(0.1129)
HH size	0.7065*	0.5350*	0.1873*	-0.1750*	-0.3726*	-0.3892*	-1.3897*
	(0.0269)	(0.0191)	(0.0205)	(0.0279)	(0.0209)	(0.0184)	(0.6136)
Age	-0.3889*	-0.2343*	-0.1138*	-0.0688*	0.1162*	0.2490*	-2.6212*
	(0.0213)	(0.0158)	(0.0184)	(0.0213)	(0.0175)	(0.0168)	(0.3152)
Employment	0.0034	-0.0098*	-0.0189*	0.0126*	0.0161*	-0.0002	-0.1140
	(0.0033)	(0.0022)	(0.0025)	(0.0032)	(0.0025)	(0.0021)	(0.0647)
Education	-0.0663*	-0.0302*	0.0345*	-0.0295*	-0.0074*	0.0334*	0.0023
	(0.0034)	(0.0022)	(0.0022)	(0.0030)	(0.0022)	(0.0018)	(0.0613)
House	-0.0248*	0.0188*	0.0558*	-0.1003*	0.0078	-0.0709*	-0.2782*
	(0.0081)	(0.0047)	(0.0057)	(0.0070)	(0.0054)	(0.0047)	(0.1068)
Single	0.1001*	0.0589*	0.0141*	-0.0561*	-0.0796*	-0.0707*	-0.4271*
	(0.0085)	(0.0062)	(0.0063)	(0.0077)	(0.0056)	(0.0050)	(0.1634)
Black	0.0224*	-0.0063*	-0.0582*	0.0319*	0.0148*	-0.0147*	-0.0028
	(0.0012)	(0.0010)	(0.0019)	(0.0009)	(0.0007)	(0.0011)	(0.0211)
Hisp	0.0140*	0.0007	-0.0036*	0.0049*	0.0050*	0.0015*	0.0219*
	(0.0006)	(0.0005)	(0.0006)	(0.0007)	(0.0005)	(0.0005)	(0.0092)
Popdensi	-0.0284*	-0.0403*	0.0032	0.0041	-0.0179*	0.0105*	0.1849*
	(0.0023)	(0.0016)	(0.0016)	(0.0023)	(0.0016)	(0.0015)	(0.0388)
AgeC6	0.0148*	0.0033*	-0.0013*	0.0073*	0.0017*	0.0015*	0.0134
	(0.0003)	(0.0003)	(0.0005)	(0.0006)	(0.0007)	(0.0006)	(0.0106)
AgeC1317	-0.0024*	0.0008	0.0052*	-0.0236*	-0.0098*	-0.0075*	0.0487*
	(0.0010)	(0.0006)	(0.0007)	(0.0019)	(0.0012)	(0.0011)	(0.0228)
	RFBO	LFBO	WHSO	RFSO	LFSO		
HH income	0.6399*	0.4860*	0.2795*	0.2536*	0.4503*		
	(0.0884)	(0.0599)	(0.0338)	(0.0236)	(0.0213)		
HH size	0.9937*	0.4682*	-0.3246*	-0.1965	-0.6767*		
	(0.2746)	(0.2209)	(0.1268)	(0.1147)	(0.0831)		
Age	-0.6132	-1.2710*	-0.9245*	-0.9620*	-0.9654*		
	(0.4762)	(0.1900)	(0.1097)	(0.0983)	(0.0774)		
Employment	-0.0484	-0.0715*	-0.0806*	-0.1112*	-0.0679*		
	(0.0399)	(0.0303)	(0.0158)	(0.0136)	(0.0102)		
Education	-0.0209	0.1079*	0.0368*	0.0977*	0.0899*		
	(0.0338)	(0.0292)	(0.0155)	(0.0131)	(0.0097)		
House	0.4806*	0.1486	-0.1821*	0.0018	-0.1028*		
	(0.2012)	(0.0872)	(0.0325)	(0.0364)	(0.0270)		
Single	0.1715	0.1334*	0.0581	-0.0120	-0.1540*		

Table 3. (Continued)

	Percentage changes in purchase probability						
	(0.0986)	(0.0677)	(0.0399)	(0.0323)	(0.0238)		
Black	-0.0257*	-0.0527*	-0.0059	-0.0006	-0.0234*		
	(0.0146)	(0.0171)	(0.0072)	(0.0057)	(0.0051)		
Hisp	-0.0034	0.0003	0.0054	0.0114*	0.0086*		
	(0.0099)	(0.0075)	(0.0033)	(0.0024)	(0.0022)		
Popdensi	0.0870*	0.0622*	0.1226*	0.0259*	0.0964*		
	(0.0405)	(0.0198)	(0.0103)	(0.0107)	(0.0079)		
AgeC6	0.0186*	0.0082	0.0419*	0.0050*	-0.0012		
	(0.0072)	(0.0043)	(0.0020)	(0.0024)	(0.0019)		
AgeC1317	-0.0040	-0.0053*	-0.0165*	-0.0095*	0.0109*		
	(0.0148)	(0.0103)	(0.0063)	(0.0050)	(0.0035)		

Source: Calculated by authors using 2007-08 Nielsen Homescan data.

Notes: The figures in each row are the percentage changes in the probability of buying each of the 12 products (in the top row) following a 1-percent increase (or for dichotomous variables from 0 to 1) in each of the household variables (in the first column). Standard errors are in parentheses and "*" indicates significant at level of 0.05 or better.

WHBC = Whole, big (1 gallon), conventional; RFBC = Reduced-fat, big, conventional; LFBC = Low-fat, big, conventional; WHSC = Whole, small (less than gallon), conventional; RFSC = Reduced-fat, small, conventional; LFSC = Low-fat, small, conventional; WHBO = Whole, big, organic; RFBO = Reduced-fat, big, organic; LFBO = Low-fat, big, organic; WHSO = Whole, small, organic; RFSO = Reduced-fat, small, organic; LFSO = Low-fat, small, organic

Low-fat milk is defined as less than 2 percent fat including skim; reduced-fat is between 2 and 3.25 percent fat; and whole is at least 3.25 percent fat.

HH = Household; Age = age of female head; Popdensi = population density of the household residential area.

Employment: = 1 if female head employed; = 0 if not

Education: = 1 if female head gained college education; = 0 if not

House: = 1 if owned house; = 0 if not

Single: = 1 if household size is 1; = 0 if not

Black: =1 if household is African American; =0 if other

Hisp: = 1 if household is Hispanic; = 0 if not

AgeC6: = 1 if presence of children 6 and below; = 0 if not

AgeC1317: = 1 if presence of children between 13 and 17; = 0 if not

Table 4. Percentage changes in purchase probability with respect to a 1-percent increase in fluid milk prices

						Percentage changes in purchase probability						
Price	WHBC	RFBC	LFBC	WHSC	RFSC	LFSC	WHBO	RFBO	LFBO	WHSO	RFSO	LFSO
WHBC	-0.6153	0.1312	0.1575	0.0649	0.1112	0.1283	0.0005	0.0009	0.0019	0.0034	0.0056	0.0099
RFBC	0.0553	-0.5140	0.1492	0.0615	0.1054	0.1216	0.0005	0.0008	0.0018	0.0032	0.0053	0.0094
LFBC	0.0534	0.1202	-0.4727	0.0595	0.1018	0.1175	0.0005	0.0008	0.0017	0.0031	0.0051	0.0090
WHSC	0.0867	0.1951	0.2341	-0.9050	0.1653	0.1908	0.0007	0.0013	0.0028	0.0051	0.0083	0.0147
RFSC	0.0826	0.1858	0.2228	0.0920	-0.7963	0.1816	0.0007	0.0012	0.0027	0.0048	0.0079	0.0140
LFSC	0.0807	0.1816	0.2187	0.0899	0.1538	-0.7543	0.0007	0.0012	0.0026	0.0047	0.0077	0.0137
WHBO	0.0917	0.2062	0.2475	0.1021	0.1747	0.2017	-1.0579	0.0013	0.0029	0.0054	0.0088	0.0155
RFBO	0.0857	0.1928	0.2314	0.0953	0.1631	0.1885	0.0007	-0.9880	0.0028	0.0050	0.0082	0.0145
LFBO	0.0852	0.1916	0.2298	0.0948	0.1623	0.1874	0.0007	0.0012	-0.9807	0.0050	0.0082	0.0145
WHSO	0.1189	0.2674	0.3209	0.1324	0.2267	0.2615	0.0010	0.0017	0.0038	-1.3659	0.0114	0.0201
RFSO	0.1174	0.2642	0.3171	0.1308	0.2239	0.2583	0.0010	0.0017	0.0038	0.0069	-1.3450	0.0199
LFSO	0.1167	0.2625	0.3150	0.1300	0.2224	0.2566	0.0010	0.0017	0.0037	0.0068	0.0111	**-1.3276**

Source: Calculated by authors using 2007-08 Nielsen Homescan data.

Notes: The figures in each row are the percentage changes in the probability of buying each of the 12 products (in the top row) following a 1-percent increase in each product's price (in the first column). All the elasticities are significant at the level of 0.05 or better. WHBC = Whole, big (1 gallon), conventional; RFBC = Reduced-fat, big, conventional; LFBC = Low-fat, big, conventional ; WHSC = Whole, small (less than gallon), conventional; RFSC = Reduced-fat, small, conventional; LFSC = Low-fat, small, conventional; WHBO = Whole, big, organic; RFBO = Reduced-fat, big, organic; LFBO = Low-fat, big, organic; WHSO = Whole, small, organic; RFSO = Reduced-fat, small, organic; LFSO = Low-fat, small, organic.

Low-fat milk is defined as less than 2 percent fat including skim; reduced-fat is between 2 and 3.25 percent fat; and whole is at least 3.25 percent fat.

On the other hand, these households may be more exposed to further income decreases and/or price increases. To the extent that they are already purchasing less expensive items, they will have less room in their budgets to further economize.

One exception is the fat content of milk. Consistent with Davis et al. (2010), we find a positive association between higher income and the probability of purchasing low-fat, conventional milk in a gallon container, which is the least expensive of all of our 12 products. Also, larger families are more likely to buy a big container of whole, conventional milk than a big container of whole, organic milk. However, household size appears to affect primarily the choice of container size. Not surprisingly, larger households tend to buy milk in larger packages.

The age of the female head of household is another important choice determinant. When people get older, they are more likely to buy reduced or low-fat conventional milk in a smaller container. Other research has shown that fluid milk consumption tends to decrease with age (e.g., Sebastian et al., 2010), suggesting that a gallon container may contain more milk than older household members can drink before it spoils. Regarding the influence of children in a household, the results show that presence of small children (6 years old or less) increases the probability of buying all types of milk besides conventional, low-fat milk in a 1-gallon container. However, the presence of teenagers between ages 13 and 17 has positive effects on the probability of buying organic, whole milk in a 1-gallon container, as well as conventional, low-fat milk in a 1-gallon container. That the effects differ depending on children's ages suggests that people may start to select different beverages in their early teenage years. Similar to past studies, we find a positive association between education and the demand for organic milk (e.g., Alviola and Capps, 2010), as well as a positive connection between education and the demand for lower fat milk products (e.g., Davis et al., 2010). Finally, when a household owns a house, it has a higher probability of buying either reduced-fat or low-fat milk in a 1-gallon container. Such households may have sufficient storage space in their homes to accommodate larger package sizes.

Price and Deal Variables

Prices and promotional deals can sway a household's choice among different milk products. Our results reveal that changing the price of any one of the 12 milk products affects the probability that a household buys that specific product (table 4). However, the magnitude of the response varies

Table 5. Percentage changes in purchase probability with respect to a 1-percent increase in use of fluid milk promotional deals

Deal	WHBC	RFBC	LFBC	WHSC	RFSC	LFSC	WHBO	RFBO	LFBO	WHSO	RFSO	LFSO
WHBC	0.1337	-0.0285	-0.0343	-0.0141	-0.0241	-0.0279	-0.0001	-0.0002	-0.0004	-0.0007	-0.0012	-0.0021
RFBC	-0.0152	0.1417	-0.0413	-0.0169	-0.0290	-0.0335	-0.0001	-0.0002	-0.0005	-0.0009	-0.0014	-0.0026
LFBC	-0.0172	-0.0386	0.1517	-0.0191	-0.0327	-0.0377	-0.0001	-0.0003	-0.0005	-0.0010	-0.0016	-0.0029
WHSC	-0.0086	-0.0194	-0.0232	0.0897	-0.0164	-0.0189	-0.0001	-0.0001	-0.0003	-0.0005	-0.0008	-0.0014
RFSC	-0.0115	-0.0259	-0.0311	-0.0127	0.1108	-0.0253	-0.0001	-0.0002	-0.0004	-0.0007	-0.0011	-0.0019
LFSC	-0.0132	-0.0298	-0.0357	-0.0147	-0.0252	0.1236	-0.0001	-0.0002	-0.0004	-0.0008	-0.0013	-0.0022
WHBO	-0.0176	-0.0397	-0.0479	-0.0198	-0.0336	-0.0390	0.2041	-0.0002	-0.0006	-0.0011	-0.0017	-0.0030
RFBO	-0.0103	-0.0233	-0.0280	-0.0115	-0.0197	-0.0227	-0.0001	0.1193	-0.0003	-0.0006	-0.0010	-0.0018
LFBO	-0.0164	-0.0369	-0.0444	-0.0182	-0.0312	-0.0361	-0.0001	-0.0002	0.1889	-0.0010	-0.0016	-0.0028
WHSO	-0.0166	-0.0372	-0.0447	-0.0184	-0.0316	-0.0365	-0.0001	-0.0002	-0.0005	0.1903	-0.0016	-0.0028
RFSO	-0.0152	-0.0343	-0.0412	-0.0170	-0.0291	-0.0336	-0.0001	-0.0002	-0.0005	-0.0009	0.1747	-0.0026
LFSO	-0.0184	-0.0414	-0.0497	-0.0205	-0.0351	-0.0405	-0.0002	-0.0003	-0.0006	-0.0011	-0.0018	0.2094

Source: Calculated by authors using 2007-08 Nielsen Homescan data.

Notes: The figures in each row are the percentage changes in the probability of buying each of the 12 products (in the top row) following a 1-percent increase in the use of deals to promote each product (in the first column). All the elasticities are significant at the level of 0.05 or better.

WHBC = Whole, big (1 gallon), conventional; RFBC = Reduced-fat, big, conventional; LFBC = Low-fat, big, conventional ; WHSC = Whole, small (less than gallon), conventional; RFSC = Reduced-fat, small, conventional; LFSC = Low-fat, small, conventional; WHBO = Whole, big, organic; RFBO = Reduced-fat, big, organic; LFBO = Low-fat, big, organic; WHSO = Whole, small, organic; RFSO = Reduced-fat, small, organic; LFSO = Low-fat, small, organic.

Low-fat milk is defined as less than 2 percent fat including skim; *reduced-fat* is between 2 and 3.25 percent fat; and *whole* is at least 3.25 percent fat.

widely. Shown in bold along the diagonal elements of table 4 are each product's own-price effects. For example, if the price of conventionally produced whole milk sold in a gallon container increases by 1 percent, holding all other prices constant, then the probability of buying this product decreases by 0.62 percent.

Own-price effects are significantly larger for organic milk products. Indeed, a 1-percent increase in the price of organically produced whole milk sold in a gallon container lowers the probability of buying this product by 1.06 percent.

That is, the change in purchase probability is proportionally greater than the percentage change in the product's own price. In terms of fat content, we see that whole milk is most sensitive to own-price changes. In terms of container size, products sold in less-than-gallon packages are more sensitive to own-price changes. In general, the change in purchase probability is larger for more expensive products.

Our results also show that households switch to less expensive products when prices rise. Shown in the off-diagonal elements in table 4 are the cross-price effects. For example, holding all other prices constant, if the price of a gallon of conventionally produced whole milk increases by 1 percent, the probability of buying a gallon of conventionally produced low-fat milk increases by 0.16 percent.

As shown in table 1, lower fat products tend to cost less than higher fat products. By contrast, an increase in the price of conventional milk sold in small containers primarily increases the probability that households buy the same type of milk in a gallon container. Finally, if the price of any one of the organic milk products increases, the probability that a household switches to conventional milk increases by more than does the probability the household buys another type of organic milk.

Our results show that promotional deals and increases in milk price have similar effects on purchase probabilities (table 5), but those effects are in opposite directions. In other words, promotional deals may work to counteract the effects of price changes.

In our analysis, an increased probability of buying one product—caused either by a change in price or the use of promotional deals—must decrease the probability of buying 1 or more of the 11 other milk products (tables 4 and 5). Indeed, the figures in each row of the 2 tables are the percentage changes in the probability of buying each of the 12 products following either a 1-percent increase in 1 product's price (table 4) or a 1-percent increase in the use of deals to promote that product (table 5). Because households must buy only 1 of the 12 products on any particular occasion when they buy milk, the figures in each row sum to zero.

Impact of Price and Income Shocks on Market Composition

In the December 2007-June 2009 recession, prices increased for fluid milk and other staples. Kumcu and Kaufman (2011) show that, during that recession, consumers reacted by looking for ways to economize. We investigate how households adjusted their choices among fluid milk products. However, because many types of price and income shocks could again occur, we use our estimated model to simulate the effects of some possible future shocks. The elasticities in tables 3-5 are best interpreted as the percentage changes in the probability of buying a particular fluid milk product following 1-percent changes in income, price, and promotional deals, as well as changes to other variables. We now use these elasticities to predict changes in households' choices among all 12 fluid milk products in selected scenarios. Consider, for example, a 1-percent price increase for all products. To begin, because of the increase in that product's own price, we note that the probability of buying conventionally produced whole milk in a gallon container would decrease by 0.62 percent. At the same time, because of increases in the prices of the other 11 products, the same purchase probability increases by 0.06 percent, 0.05 percent, 0.09 percent, 0.08 percent, and so on. In total, summing the own-price and 11 cross-price effects in the first column of table 4, we find that the probability of buying conventionally produced whole milk in a gallon container increases by about 0.36 percent (table 6). Next, given the product's baseline market share of 8.8 percent (table 1), we estimate its new market share under the alternative scenario of a 1-percent general price increase. Though the new market share is very slightly higher, it is still roughly less than 9 percent (i.e., 0.088 + (0.0036 x 0.088)). After repeating this same series of steps for the other 11 products, we can aggregate over our predictions for each individual product to further estimate the re-division of fluid milk sales categorized by fat content, method of production, and package size. This would complete simulation results for a 1-percent increase in all fluid milk prices. Notably, we must repeat all calculations for other chosen scenarios. The process of calculating each product's new market share and aggregating over the predictions for all 12 products to estimate the re-division of the market categorized along three dimensions is a nonlinear process. For example, the impact of 10-percent price increase is not simply 10 times the impact of a 1-percent price increase. Finally, predictions derived for each scenario can be compared against the baseline scenario. Of all fluid milk purchased by U.S. households in 2007-08, 17 percent was whole, 47 percent was low-fat, and 36 percent was reduced-fat. Gallon packages accounted for about 58 percent of all purchases. Organic products represented about 3 percent of all sales. The results of the simulations are shown in tables 6 and 7. Some of the scenarios are also provided in figure 1.

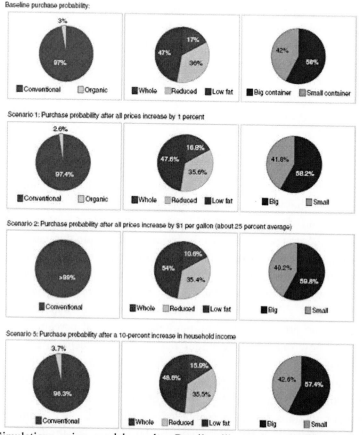

Note: Simulations using model results. Retail milk products divided along three dimensions including method of production (organic and conventional), fat content (low-fat, reduced-fat, and whole), and container size (gallon or small-sized container). Source: Calculated by authors using 2007-08 Nielsen Homescan data.

Figure 1. Simulation results for several scenarios.

Retail fluid milk prices tend to be volatile, as they fluctuate with prices that dairy farmers receive for milk (Stewart and Blayney, 2011). We examined monthly retail milk prices between 2000 and 2011[9] and find that retail prices typically change by 1 to 2 percent per month. However, retail prices are also highly cyclical. They can trend upward or downward for extended periods of time.

The price of a gallon of fluid milk at the high and low points of a cycle can differ by 25 percent or more. To begin, in scenario 1 (fig. 1), we report the effects of a 1-percent increase in price for all milk products. Not surprisingly, as shown in the first two columns of numbers in tables 6 and 7 as well as in fig. 1, a 1-percent change in price has only small impacts on the composition of the fluid milk market.

The second scenario (table 7 and fig. 1) simulates the market share changes if prices for all 12 milk products rose, as in 2007-08. In those years, higher prices received by farmers for milk pushed retail prices for fluid milk as much as 25 percent higher (e.g., Stewart and Blayney, 2011). Although small shocks may have only small effects on the market, could such a large shock to prices motivate people to substitute, in significant quantities, less expensive products like conventional milk for more expensive products like organic milk?

The elasticities are substantially less accurate when used to simulate much larger shocks, but may still serve as a very general indicator of whether market shares are likely to change only a little or a lot.

Following the same procedure outlined above, we find that milk price increases of $1 per gallon (approximately 25 percent) for all 12 products could slow growth in sales of organic milk, just as rising prices and the recession did between 2007 and 2009.

By the simulation, the magnitude of the loss in organic market share could nearly equal the overall 2007-08 organic market share of 2 to 3 percent. We again caution that this estimate does not precisely measure the likely changes in market shares. However, the simulation does indicate that the impact on the organic market would be substantial. Likewise, the purchase probabilities decrease from 17 to 10.6 percent for whole milk; decrease from 36 to 35.4 percent for reduced-fat milk; and increase from 47 to 54 percent for low-fat milk. The probability of purchasing milk in a small container decreases from 42 to 40.2 percent, while the probability of buying it in a big container increases from 58 to 59.8 percent.

Table 6. Percentage changes in probability of purchasing fluid milk with respect to a 1-percent change in household variables

| | 1-percent increase of all milk prices | 1-percent increase of organic milk prices | Percentage changes in purchase probability | | | | | |
			$1 increase of all milk prices	1-percent increase of all milk deal	1-percent increase of organic milk deal	1-percent increase of income	1-person increase of hhsize	1-year increase of age
WHBC	0.3590	0.6156	0.7520	-0.0400	-0.5220	-0.2315	0.3168	-0.0069
RFBC	1.6846	1.3847	25.2530	-1.3428	-1.1759	-0.1005	0.2399	-0.0042
LFBC	2.1713	1.6617	34.1143	-1.8164	-1.4140	0.0588	0.0840	-0.0020
WHSC	0.1482	0.6854	2.9480	-0.1579	-0.5823	-0.0941	-0.0785	-0.0012
RFSC	1.0143	1.1731	18.4712	-0.9902	-0.9962	-0.0155	-0.1671	0.0021
LFSC	1.3395	1.3540	24.2571	-1.2984	-1.1512	0.1063	-0.1745	0.0044
WHBO	-1.0499	-1.0535	-18.7373	1.0028	1.0070	0.0410	-0.6232	-0.0468
RFBO	-0.9742	-0.9804	-18.5919	1.0062	1.0140	0.6399	0.4456	-0.0110
LFBO	-0.9502	-0.9637	-18.2438	0.9742	0.9910	0.4860	0.2100	-0.0227
WHSO	-1.3125	-1.3368	-17.7120	0.9449	0.9754	0.2795	-0.1456	-0.0165
RFSO	-1.2574	-1.2973	-16.9845	0.8955	0.9447	0.2536	-0.0881	-0.0172
LFSO	-1.1724	-1.2431	-15.5195	0.8218	0.9085	0.4503	-0.3035	-0.0172
Conventional	6.7167	6.8746	105.79	-5.6455	-5.8410	-0.2765	0.2206	-0.0079
Organic	-6.7167	-6.8746	-105.79	5.6455	5.8410	2.1503	-0.5048	-0.1314
Total	0	0	0	0	0	1.8738	-0.2842	-0.1393

Source: Calculated by authors using 2007-08 Nielsen Homescan data.

Note: First column of the table indicates the type of milk product, as follows: WHBC = Whole, big (1 gallon), conventional; RFBC = Reduced-fat, big, conventional; LFBC = Low-fat, big, conventional; WHSC = Whole, small (less than gallon), conventional; RFSC = Reduced-fat, small, conventional; LFSC = Low-fat, small, conventional; WHBO = Whole, big, organic; RFBO = Reduced-fat, big, organic; LFBO = Low-fat, big, organic; WHSO = Whole, small, organic; RFSO = Reduced-fat, small, organic; LFSO = Low-fat, small, organic

Low-fat milk is defined as less than 2 percent fat including skim; reduced-fat is between 2 and 3.25 percent fat; and whole is at least 3.25 percent fat.

Table 7. Simulation results for purchase probability

	Baseline	Scenario 1 1-percent increase of all milk prices	Scenario 2 $1 increase of all milk prices	Scenario 3 1-percent increase of organic milk prices	Scenario 4 10-percent increase of all milk deals	Scenario 5 10-percent increase of income	Scenario 6 1-person increase of hhsize	Scenario 7 1-year increase of age
					Purchase probability			
Conventional	97.0	97.4	100	97.4	90.0	96.3	97.0	97.0
Organic	3.0	2.6	<1	2.6	10.0	3.7	3.0	3.0
1-gallon container	58.0	58.2	59.8	57.9	56.5	57.4	58.1	57.6
Small container	42.0	41.8	40.2	42.1	43.5	42.6	41.9	42.4
Whole	17.0	16.8	10.6	17.0	21.2	15.9	17.2	17.2
Reduced fat	36.0	35.6	35.4	35.6	35.8	35.5	35.7	35.6
Low fat	47.0	47.6	54.0	47.4	43.0	48.6	47.1	47.2
Total	100	100	100	100	100	100	100	100

Source: Calculated by authors using 2007-08 Nielsen Homescan data.

In the third scenario (table 7 and fig. 1), we consider the possibility that prices for organic and conventional milk products need not move together. Costs for feed and other inputs used exclusively by organic dairy farming could rise faster or slower than costs for inputs used by conventional dairy farmers. That may have been the case in 2011. Neuman (2011) reports that costs for organic farmers rose faster that year.

For the simulation, we consider the effect of a 1-percent increase in the price of the six organic products while holding constant prices for the six conventional products.

Interestingly, the change in purchase probability for organic products is not much larger than the predicted impact of a 1-percent increase in the price of all milk products. This difference may reflect the fact that sales of organic products are more sensitive to price changes than sales of conventional products.

Promotional deals and price increases similarly affect a household's choice among milk products, although in opposite directions. To simulate the impact of promotional deals, we consider a 10-percent increase in promotions for all 12 milk products in scenario 4. Large increases in the probability of buying organic milk occur. In fact, the purchase probability for any one of the six organic milk products increases from 3 percent in the baseline scenario to 10.5 percent. This finding underscores the sensitivity of organic milk sales to both retail prices and the use of promotional deals.

For the final simulation, we consider the effects on market composition of shocks to income, as well as changes in household size and age. As shown in table 3, the effects of the latter two demographic variables are small but statistically significant. Rising income increases the probability of purchasing lower fat and organic products.

A 10-percent increase in household income raises the probability of purchasing organic milk from 3 to 3.7 percent. A 10-percent increase in income also lowers the probabilities of purchasing whole milk from 17 to 15.9 percent and reduced-fat milk from 36 to 35.5 percent.

The probablility of buying low-fat milk increases from 47 to 48.6 percent. Only small changes occur to a household's choice among products in different container sizes. In contrast to household income changes, changes in household size and age have no effect on the probabilities of purchasing conventional and organic milk, but do affect substantially choice of container size (table 7).

CONCLUSION

During the December 2007 to June 2009 recession, many U.S. household experienced a decrease in income. In addition, food prices rose 4 percent in 2007 and 5.5 percent in 2008 before moderating to 1.8 percent in 2009. In this study, we examine some of the strategies that households use to stretch their food dollar in response to income and price shocks.

In particular, we focus on how they adjust their choice among fluid milk products categorized along three dimensions: three levels of fat content, two levels of package size, and organic versus conventionally produced products. Though fluid milk is a staple of the American diet, most Americans aged 4 and over do not consume enough dairy products.

Among the key results, households experiencing an income decrease substitute less expensive products for more expensive ones. The demand for organic milk is particularly sensitive to changes in income. Also, price fluctuations can influence a household's fluid milk purchases. In the recent past, retail milk prices have fluctuated by as much as 25 percent. A price increase of this magnitude has little impact on whether a household chooses to buy fluid milk in a 1-gallon or smaller sized container. It would decrease the probability that a household buys low-fat milk from 47 to 53.9 percent. Moreover, a 25-percent increase in retail fluid milk prices is large enough to reduce growth in sales of organic milk, as happened recently in 2007-08.

APPENDIX I: THE SPECIFICATION OF THE HOUSEHOLD LOYALTY VARIABLE (L_{IJT})

Households are heterogeneous with their own specific, seemingly idiosyncratic preferences among the products available at retail stores. These preferences may stay the same over time, but may also change based on households' purchase experience. For example, suppose that household A derives greater utility from product i than does household B at time t. If the two households face the same price and other variables are constant, the relative probability between the two households (i.e., the purchase probability for product i by household A is bigger than the one for household B) tends to remain the same for future purchases. However, if the households each gain more and more experience purchasing product i, they may adjust their purchase preferences over time, and the relative purchase probability for product i between the two households could be reversed. Fader and Lattin (1993) also point out that preferences can change with sudden, unforeseen occurrences. Household-specific preferences for given products are unobservable and are associated with household-specific demographic variables, as well as purchase experience. They are the household's intrinsic loyalty to the products it purchases. They are different from the observed purchase probabilities, which also depend on prices, promotional deals, and other marketing variables.

In this study, we follow Fader and Lattin (1993) and Dong and Stewart (2012) to define the loyalty probability $_{(Lijt)}$ in equation (1) using the Dirichlet distribution and assume that the likelihood of a nonstationary change (a renewal) in the product loyalty probabilities for a given household between purchase occasions can be described by a Bernouli distribution. We then derive the expected product loyalty probabilities (i.e., the Dirichlet posterior probabilities) from the observed choice behavior of the household and use these posterior probabilities to form the basis of $Lijt$.

Suppose that there are J products to choose from for a given household to buy milk at time t. Absent any information on households' income and demographic characteristics or their prior purchase history, we assume the prior probabilities of choosing each of the J products, $\rho_1, \rho_2 \ldots, \rho_j$, follow a Dirichlet distribution with parameters $\theta_1, \theta_2 \ldots, \theta_j$. The *pdf* of the Dirichlet distribution is

$$D(\rho_1, \rho_2 \cdots, \rho_j) = \frac{\Gamma(\theta_1 + \theta_2 + \cdots + \theta_j)}{\Gamma(\theta_1)\Gamma(\theta_2)\cdots\Gamma(\theta_j)} \rho_1^{\theta_1-1} \rho_2^{\theta_2-1} \cdots \rho_j^{\theta_j-1}$$

(A1)

where $\Gamma(\cdot)$ is the gamma function, and all θs are positive. From equation (A1) we know

$$E(\rho_j) = \frac{\theta_j}{\sum_{i=1}^{j} \theta_i}$$

(A2)

where $E(.)$ is expectation operation.

The θs are product-specific parameters that indicate the relative level of a household's preference for each product in the absence of any other information. Thus, equation (A2) gives the household initial choice (loyalty) probabilities to each of the products. However, according to Bayes Theorem, the probabilities can be updated at time t using a household's observed product choice history for milk purchases from time 1 through time $t - 1$, if these data are available. If we use y_{ijr} to represent household i's choice history, and define that y_{ijr} equals 1 if household i purchased product j at time r and equals zero otherwise, then we can update the probabilities given by equation (A1) using a new Dirichlet distribution with the parameters:

$$\theta_1 + \sum_{r=1}^{t-1} y_{i1r}, \theta_2 + \sum_{r=1}^{t-1} y_{i2r}, \cdots, \theta_J + \sum_{r=1}^{t-1} y_{iJr}$$

Equation (A2) is updated for the new expected probability given the purchase history data, as the following:

$$E(\rho_{ijt} \mid y_{ijr}) = \frac{\theta_j + \sum_{r=1}^{t-1} y_{ijr}}{\sum_{l=1}^{J} \theta_l + t - 1}, \tag{A3}$$

where $t - 1$ is the total number of food purchases through time $t -1$ by household i.

The model allows for household heterogeneity through $\sum_{r=1}^{t-1} y_{ijr}$, the observed household purchase history. To further capture heterogeneity caused by household demographics, we follow Dong and Stewart (2012) to extend the model through the parameterization of θ_j, using the vector of household variables, Z_{it}:

$$\theta_{ijt} = e^{\gamma_{0j} + \gamma_{1j} Z_{it}}, \tag{A4}$$

where the parameters γ_{0j} and γ_{1j} are unique to each product. Age, income, household size, and other variables may be included in Z_{it} as past studies and economic theory suggest. The exponential specification of equation (A4) is to guarantee that θ_{ijt} is positive.

To allow for any sudden, unforeseen occurrences that might influence a household's product choices (for example, the entry and exit of a new brand, a new advertising campaign), we expand the Dirichlet probability formulation as a nonstationary process.

Nonstationarity in the Dirichlet choice model is assumed to be a renewal process. This renewal process may be described as follows: For any given time (purchase occasion), the household may renew its choice or loyalty probability because of sudden or unforeseen reasons with a probability of $1 - \lambda$, where $0 \leq \lambda \leq 1$. As described by Fader and Lattin (1993), each renewal constitutes a new draw from the original Dirichlet distribution, restarts the purchase history from the renewal point until the next renewal, and is independent of previous renewals. Thus, the probability of k purchases elapsing without renewal since the last renewal is $(1 - \lambda) \lambda^k$, which is geometrically distributed, with λ being constant across households.

If a sudden, unforeseen event has changed a household's product choices, then only its behavior since that event provides useful information for predicting its current behavior. Given the nonstationary Dirichlet choice process for household i with an observed purchase history from occasions 1 to $t - 1$, the expected loyalty probability for product j at time t is given by

$$E(\rho_{ijt} \mid y_{ijr}) = \sum_{k=0}^{t-1} E(\rho_{ijt} \mid k) \cdot \delta_k,$$

(A5)

with

$$E(\rho_{ijt} \mid k) = \frac{\theta_{ijt} + \sum_{r=t-k}^{t-1} y_{ijr}}{\sum_{l=1}^{j} \theta_{ilt} + k},$$

(A6)

and

$$(A7) \quad \delta_k = (1 - \lambda)\lambda^k,$$

(A7)

where $k = 0, 1, \ldots, t-1$; δ_k is the probability of k purchases elapsing without renewal since the last renewal; and y_{ijr} equals one if household i purchased product j at time r, and equals zero otherwise. When $k = 0$, we define. θ_{ijt} is given in equation (A4), and λ is a parameter.

Allowing for household heterogeneity through both demographics and past purchase history, as well as possible nonstationarity, the specification of the household heterogeneity variable becomes

$$L_{ijt} = E(\rho_{ijt} \mid y_{ijr}) = \sum_{k=0}^{t-2} \varphi_{ijk}\delta_k + \varphi_{ijt-1}(1 - \sum_{k=0}^{t-2} \delta_k)$$

(A8)

based on equation (A5), with $\varphi_{ijk} = E(\rho_{ijt} \mid k)$ as given in equation (A6) and δ_k as given in equation (A7).

APPENDIX II: ESTIMATION RESULTS

Our data appear to fit the model well. From the appendix table, we see that the predicted purchase probabilities for the 12 milk products are quite consistent with the data provided in table 1. Also, prices and promotional deals are significant at the 1-percent level. These marketing variables directly affect product choices and have the expected signs. Notably, given the specification of household utility in equation (1), these variables have the same coefficient (β) for all milk products. However, prices and promotions will still have different effects on the purchase probabilities for each product, in accordance with equation (4) for the variables' marginal effects (Dong and Stewart, 2012). The product-specific constants and some of the seasonal dummy variables are also significant at the 1-percent level. The constant and the coefficient on the seasonal dummy variable for the product *conventional, whole milk in a gallon container* were restricted to zero for the purpose of normalization, so that the values for all other products are relative to the value of this product. From equation (1), we see that household variables indirectly influence milk product choices through the household loyalty variable. Many of these variables are significant at the 1-percent level, including income, household size, age, and house ownership, among others. The effects of these variables on the purchase probabilities vary among milk products. Also significant is λ, the nonstationary probability associated with the loyalty variable. It indicates how often a household's product choices are influenced by sudden, unforeseen occurrences, such as a new promotional marketing campaign. A value near one indicates that such events rarely occurred.

Appendix Table: Model estimates

Variable	WHBC	RFBC	LFBC	WHSC	RFSC	LFSC
Probability:	0.0866	0.1948	0.2338	0.0964	0.1651	0.1905
Household Variables: Intercept	3.6185* (0.1242)	2.2020* (0.1115)	-3.0533* (0.1273)	-0.4436* (0.1474)	-2.416* (0.1252)	-5.6751* (0.1178)
Log HH income	-0.4046* (0.0114)	-0.2107* (0.0089)	0.1214* (0.0107)	-0.1788* (0.0119)	-0.0355* (0.0099)	0.2278* (0.0091)
Inverse HHsize	-1.8928* (0.0833)	-1.7144* (0.0714)	-0.5351* (0.0791)	0.7059* (0.0980)	1.5431* (0.0870)	1.6437* (0.0790)
Age	-0.0133* (0.0007)	-0.0096* (0.0006)	-0.0052* (0.0008)	-0.0032* (0.0008)	0.0035* (0.0007)	0.0089* (0.0007)
Employment:	0.0071 (0.0144)	-0.0567* (0.0121)	-0.1055* (0.0142)	0.0503* (0.0155)	0.0749* (0.0141)	-0.0095 (0.0126)
Education	-0.2654* (0.0148)	-0.1322* (0.0122)	0.2160* (0.0136)	-0.1185* (0.0145)	-0.0176 (0.0129)	0.2174* (0.0118)
House	-0.0707* (0.0186)	0.0317* (0.0136)	0.1302* (0.0168)	-0.2509* (0.0173)	0.0023 (0.0159)	-0.2107* (0.0139)
Single	0.4248* (0.0507)	0.2113* (0.0420)	0.0696 (0.0449)	-0.5438* (0.0552)	-0.7905* (0.0482)	-0.7368* (0.0439)
Black	0.5798* (0.0267)	0.0029 (0.0230)	-0.9382* (0.0356)	0.8941* (0.0258)	0.5029* (0.0189)	-0.1755* (0.0242)
Hisp	0.6030* (0.0226)	0.1193* (0.0240)	-0.0664* (0.0267)	0.2726* (0.0282)	0.3066* (0.0223)	0.1491* (0.0229)
Popdensi	-0.0570* (0.0043)	-0.0923* (0.0037)	-0.0011 (0.0038)	0.0002 (0.0047)	-0.0466* (0.0037)	0.0147* (0.0037)
AgeC6	1.0973* (0.0195)	0.4731* (0.0242)	0.1451* (0.0329)	0.5987* (0.0355)	0.2941* (0.0391)	0.2787* (0.0314)
AgeC1317	-0.0661* (0.0204)	-0.0007 (0.0208)	0.1191* (0.0225)	-0.4599* (0.0359)	-0.2199* (0.0267)	-0.1733* (0.0230)
Marketing variables and Constant	other parameters: 0	-0.0004 (0.0133)	0.1521* (0.0148)	0.2106* (0.0371)	0.1712* (0.0324)	0.2630* (0.0310)
Spring	0	-0.0548* (0.0184)	-0.1272* (0.0203)	0.1455* (0.0198)	0.1378* (0.0200)	0.0953* (0.0207)
Summer	0	-0.0155 (0.0205)	-0.1310* (0.0230)	0.1678* (0.0223)	0.1950* (0.0227)	0.0937* (0.0235)
Fall	0	-0.0347 (0.0278)	-0.2012* (0.0304)	0.1157* (0.0288)	0.0713* (0.0297)	-0.0573 (0.0309)
Milk price	-0.1888* (0.0205)					
Milk deal	1.0121* (0.0724)					
	0.9963*					

Variable	WHBC	RFBC	LFBC	WHSC	RFSC	LFSC
	(0.0110)					
Log likelihood	-479,127.99					
Variable	WHBO	RFBO	LFBO	WHSO	RLSO	LFSO
Probability:	0.0007	0.0013	0.0028	0.0051	0.0083	0.0146
Household Variables: Intercept	-5.9509* (2.1401)	-15.5443* (1.5161)	-11.9883* (1.0309)	-9.7030* (0.5970)	-7.7794* (0.4234)	-11.992* (0.3630)
Log HH income	0.0577 (0.1650)	0.9360* (0.1297)	0.7122* (0.0882)	0.4110* (0.0501)	0.3762* (0.0354)	0.6759* (0.0323)
Inverse HHsize	3.6611* (1.5713)	-2.4464* (0.7054)	-1.0996* (0.5690)	-0.9458* (0.3291)	0.6192* (0.3008)	1.8930* (0.2208)
Age	-0.0696* (0.0083)	-0.0169 (0.0126)	-0.0344* (0.0050)	-0.0253* (0.0029)	-0.0266 (0.0026)	-0.0269* (0.0021)
Employment:	-0.4180 (0.2336)	-0.1816 (0.1446)	-0.2660* (0.1108)	-0.3007* (0.0578)	-0.4168* (0.0502)	-0.2593* (0.0381)
Education	0.0255 (0.2306)	-0.0622 (0.1279)	0.4270* (0.1113)	0.1577* (0.0593)	0.3945* (0.0509)	0.3707* (0.0383)
House	-0.5252* (0.1961)	0.8713* (0.3712)	0.2600 (0.1615)	-0.3529* (0.0605)	-0.0114 (0.0685)	-0.2094* (0.0515)
Single	-2.3133* (0.8327)	0.7376 (0.5038)	0.5435 (0.3463)	0.1598 (0.2063)	-0.2024 (0.1682)	-0.9503* (0.1261)
Black	0.0636* (0.3374)	-0.3034 (0.2339)	-0.7337* (0.2737)	0.0149 (0.1175)	0.1004 (0.0942)	-0.2725* (0.0832)
Hisp	0.7175* (0.2728)	-0.0326 (0.2927)	0.0767 (0.2233)	0.2317* (0.1000)	0.4140* (0.0745)	0.3357* (0.0692)
Popdensi	0.2668* (0.0574)	0.1226* (0.0601)	0.0861* (0.0295)	0.1769* (0.0154)	0.0325* (0.0162)	0.1403* (0.0120)
AgeC6	0.7192 (0.4347)	0.9457* (0.3012)	0.5158* (0.1812)	1.9312* (0.0835)	0.3871* (0.1005)	0.1274 (0.0815)
AgeC1317	0.7440* (0.3565)	-0.0796 (0.2331)	-0.1002 (0.1629)	-0.2785* (0.0993)	-0.1682* (0.0798)	0.1587* (0.0561)
Marketing variables and Constant	other parameters: -0.6639* (0.1280)	-0.5398* (0.0699)	-0.2341* (0.0632)	0.3530* (0.0814)	0.2164* (0.0762)	0.4907* (0.0722)
Spring	0.2284 (0.1432)	-0.0776 (0.0999)	-0.0347 (0.0835)	0.2897* (0.0670)	0.3056* (0.0510)	0.1197* (0.0434)
Summer	0.3212* (0.1396)	0.2462* (0.1030)	0.2518* (0.0895)	0.2195* (0.0752)	0.3821* (0.0586)	0.1632* (0.0478)
Fall	0.9846* (0.1496)	1.1154* (0.1095)	0.6669* (0.1090)	0.2169* (0.0905)	0.4104* (0.0746)	0.1006 (0.0625)
Milk price	-0.1888* (0.0205)					
Milk deal	1.0121* (0.0724)					
	0.9963* (0.0110)					
Variable	WHBO	RFBO	LFBO	WHSO	RLSO	LFSO
Log likelihood	-479,127.99					

Source: Calculated by authors using 2007-08 Nielsen Homescan data. Notes: Standard errors are in parentheses. The constant and the coefficient of grocery stores in the marketing variables are constrained to be zero. "*"indicates significant at level of 0.05 or better.

WHBC = Whole, big (1 gallon), conventional; RFBC = Reduced-fat, big, conventional; LFBC = Low-fat, big, conventional ; WHSC = Whole, small (less than gallon), conventional; RFSC = Reduced-fat, small, conventional; LFSC = Low-fat, small, conventional; WHBO = Whole, big, organic; RFBO = Reduced-fat, big, organic; LFBO = Low-fat, big, organic; WHSO = Whole, small, organic; RFSO = Reduced-fat, small, organic; LFSO = Low-fat, small, organic. Low-fat milk is defined as less than 2 percent fat including skim; reduced fat is between 2 and 3.25 percent fat; and whole is at least 3.25 percent fat. HH = Household; Age = age of female head; Popdensi = population density of the household residential area. Employment: = 1 if female head employed, = 0 if not; Education: = 1 if female head gained college education, = 0 if not; House: = 1 if owned house, = 0 if not; Single: = 1 if household size is 1, = 0 if not; Black: =1 if household is African American, =0 if other; Hisp: = 1 if household is Hispanic, = 0 if not; AgeC6: = 1 if presence of children 6 and below, = 0 if not; AgeC1317: = 1 if presence of children between 13 and 17, = 0 if not.

ACKNOWLEDGMENTS

The authors extend their thanks for helpful comments to Tirtha Dhar, Professor, University of British Columbia; Kristin Kiesel, Professor, California State University Sacramento, and Economic Research Service colleagues William Hahn and Donald Blayney. We also thank Maria Williams for editorial expertise and Curtia Taylor for the design.

REFERENCES

Alviola, P. and O. Capps, Jr. (2010). "Household Demand Analysis of Organic and Conventional Fluid Milk in the United States Based on the 2004 Nielsen Homescan Panel," *Agribusiness* 26(3): 369-388.

Andreyeva, T., M. Long, and K. Brownell (2010). "The Impact of Food Prices on Consumption: A Systematic Review of Research on the Price Elasticity of Demand for Food," *American Journal of Public Health* 100(2): 216-222.

Cornick, J., T. Cox, and B. Gould (1994). "Fluid Milk Purchases: A Multivariate Tobit Analysis," *American Journal of Agricultural Economics* 76(1): 74-82.

Davis C., D. Dong, D. Blayney, and A. Owens (2010). *An Analysis of U.S. Household Dairy Demand*, TB-1928, U.S. Department of Agriculture Economic Research Service. Available at: http://www.ers.usda.gov/ publications/tb1928/ tb1928.pdf .

DeNavas-Walt, C., B. Proctor, and J. Smith (2011). *Income, Poverty, and Health Insurance Coverage in the United States: 2010*. Current Population Reports P60-239. Washington, DC: US Census Bureau. Available at: http://www.census. gov/prod/2011pubs/p60-239.pdf.

Dhar, T. and J. Foltz (2005). "Milk by Any Other Name...Consumer Benefits from Labeled Milk," *American Journal of Agricultural Economics* 87(1): 214-228.

Dong, D. and H. Stewart (2012). "Modeling a Household's Choice Among Food Store Types," *American Journal of Agricultural Economics* 94(1): 702-717.

Dube, J. (2004). "Multiple Discreteness and Product Differentiating: Demand for Carbonated Soft Drinks," *Marketing Science*, 21 (1): 66-81.

Dupuis, E. (2000). "Not In My Body: rBGH and The Rise of Organic Milk." *Agriculture and Human Values* 17: 285-295.

Einav, L., E. Leibtag, and A. Nevo (2008). *On the Accuracy of Nielsen Homescan Data*. ERR No. 69. Washington, DC: US Department of Agriculture Economic Research Service. Available at: http://www.ers. usda.gov/Publications/ERR69/ ERR69.pdf

Fader, P. S., and J. M. Lattin (1993). "Accounting for Heterogeneity and Nonstationarity in a Cross-Sectional Model of Consumer Purchase Behavior," *Marketing Science*, 12 (Summer): 304-317.

Guadagni, P. M. and J. D. C. Little (1983). "A Logit Model of Brand Choice Calibrated on Scanner Data," *Marketing Science*, 2 (Summer): 203-238.

Hausman, J. and D. McFadden (1984). "Specification Tests for the Multinomial Logit Model," *Econometrica*, 52 (5): 1219-1240.

Kiesel, K. and S. Villas-Boas (2007). "Got Organic Milk? Consumer Valuations of Milk Labels after the Implementation of the USDA Organic Seal," *Journal of Agricultural & Food Industrial Organization* 5(4).

Kumcu, A. and P. Kaufman (2011). "Food Spending Adjustments During Recessionary Times," *Amber Waves* 9(3). Available at: http://www.ers.usda.gov/ AmberWaves/September11/

Leibtag, E. and P. Kaufman (2003). *Exploring Food Purchase Behavior of Low-Income Households.* AIB No. 747-07. Washington, DC: U.S. Department of Agriculture, Economic Research Service. Available at: http://ers.usda.gov/publications/aib747/aib74707.pdf

McBride, W. and C. Greene (2009). *Characteristics, Costs, and Issues for Organic Dairy Farming.* ERR No. 82. Washington, DC: U.S. Department of Agriculture, Economic Research Service. Available at: http://www.ers.usda.gov/Publications/ ERR82/ERR82.pdf

Neuman, W. (2011). "As Supply Dwindles, Organic Milk Gets Popular," *New York Times* December 30, 2011.

Rao, R.C. (1973). *Linear Statistical Inference and Its Applications.* Wiley, New York.

Sebastian R., Goldman J., Wilkinson Enns C., and LaComb R. (2010). *Fluid Milk Consumption in the United States: What We Eat In America, NHANES 2005-2006.* Data Brief No. 3. Beltsville, MD: U.S. Department of Agriculture, Agricultural Research Service, Food Surveys Research Group, Beltsville Human Nutrition Research Center. Available at: http://ars.usda.gov/Services/docs.htm?docid=19476 .

Smith, T., C. Huang, and B. Lin (2009). "Estimating Organic Premiums in the US Fluid Milk Market," *Renewable Agriculture and Food Systems* 24(3): 197-204.

Stewart, H. and D. Blayney (2011). "Retail Dairy Prices Fluctuate with the Farm Value of Milk," *Agricultural and Resource Economics Review* 40(1): 201-217.

U.S. Department of Agriculture, Agricultural Marketing Service (2012). Dairy Programs. Available at http://www.ams.usda.gov/AMSv1.0/ DairyLanding Page.

U.S. Department of Agriculture, Economic Research Service (2012). Loss-Adjusted Food Availability. Available at http://www.ers.usda.gov/Data/ FoodConsumption/ FoodGuideIndex.htm/.

U.S. Department of Commerce, Bureau of Labor Statistics (2012). *CPI Databases. Consumer Price Index.* Data available online: http://www.bls. gov/cpi/

U.S. Department of Agriculture and U.S. Department of Health and Human Services (2010). *Dietary Guidelines for Americans, 2010,* 7th ed. Washington, DC, December. Available at http://www.cnpp.usda.gov/ dietary guidelines. htm

End Notes

[1] Based on data provided by the U.S. Census Bureau. See DeNavas-Walt et al. (2011).

[2] Based on the Consumer Price Index (U.S. city average) as reported by the Bureau of Labor Statistics (2012).

[3] Based on the Consumer Price Index (U.S. city average) as reported by the Bureau of Labor Statistics (2012).

[4] Through its administration of Federal milk marketing orders, the USDA Agricultural Marketing Service (AMS) generates data on milk supplies, utilization, sales, plant prices, over-order payments, and retail prices for packaged milk. See USDA/AMS (2012).

[5] The Dietary Guidelines for Americans is issued by the USDA and the U.S. Department of Health and Human Services to provide evidence-based nutrition information and advice for people age 2 and older. It also serves as the basis for Federal food and nutrition education programs.

[6] Low-fat milk is defined as less than 2 percent fat including skim; reduced-fat is between 2 and 3.25 percent fat; and whole is at least 3.25 percent fat.

[7] For each given date, the prices for each of the 12 products are the average prices across households that purchased the products on that date. If no households purchased any of the 12 products on that particular date, we instead use that week's average prices.

[8] See USDA Agricultural Marketing Service (AMS) (2012).

[9] Monthly retail prices for conventional whole and conventional reduced-fat milk published by the USDA AMS were examined. See AMS (2012).

In: Milk Consumption
Editor: Francisco Paul Buren

ISBN: 978-1-62948-008-4
© 2013 Nova Science Publishers, Inc.

Chapter 3

AN ANALYSIS OF U.S. HOUSEHOLD DAIRY DEMAND*

Christopher G. Davis, Diansheng Dong, Don P. Blayney and Ashley Owens[†]

ABSTRACT

This report examines retail purchase data for 12 dairy products and margarine from the Nielsen 2007 Homescan data. Selected demographic and socioeconomic variables included in the Nielsen data are analyzed for their effects on aggregate demand and expenditure elasticities for the selected products. A censored demand system is used to derive the demand elasticities. The resulting estimates revealed that the magnitudes of 10 of the 13 own-price elasticities have absolute values greater than 1; substitute relationships are found among most dairy categories; expenditure elasticities are 1 or greater for 7 of the 13 products; and demographic and socioeconomic variables are statistically significant contributors to dairy demand.

Keywords: Butter, cheese, censored demand, elasticities, bulk ice cream, margarine, milk, Nielsen Homescan data, yogurt

---

[*] This is an edited, reformatted and augmented edition of a United States Department of Agriculture Technical Bulletin, Number 1928, dated December 2010.
[†] Ashley Owens was a student intern at Economic Research Service during the time that this study was in progress.

ACKNOWLEDGMENTS

The authors extend their thanks for helpful comments from Economic Research Service colleagues Daniel Pick, Richard Stillman, Rachel Johnson, William Hahn, and Abebayehu Tegene. They are also appreciative of the contributions of Courtney Knauth, editor, and Curtia Taylor, designer, in preparing the report for publication.

SUMMARY

What Is the Issue?

The measurement of the economic effects of food prices and consumer incomes on the demand for foods derived from agricultural products is important in economic analysis. Consumers allocate spending among a wide array of competing products sold at retail outlets across the country. In this technical study, the authors estimate how fluctuation in prices and household expenditures, as well as a number of demographic characteristics, affect household demand for 12 dairy products and margarine. These empirical estimates offer a glimpse of relationships among the 13 product categories—including ways that consumers use some of the products together or inter-changeably—which are of interest to many in the U.S. dairy industry.

What Did the Study Find?

Using a censored demand system and Nielsen Homescan data for purchase of items in the 13 categories, the authors estimated two types of elasticities: price and expenditure. The effects of selected demographic variables, based on characteristics such as household size and composition, educational level and ethnicity of household head, regional location, and household income, are also analyzed. The analysts found that:

- Ten of the 13 products have negative own-price elasticities with absolute values greater than 1.
- Strong substitution relationships exist among most dairy product categories.

- All of the expenditure elasticities are statistically significant and positive. Changes in the overall household dairy expenditure have the largest effect on purchases of reduced-fat milk, canned milk, bulk ice cream, refrigerated and frozen yogurts, natural cheese, and cottage cheese.
- Although the influence of most demographic variables is relatively small, some of them do have statistically significant effects on consumer purchases of dairy products:
  - Single-person households and households headed by a college-educated woman have a positive, statistically significant influence on the purchase of refrigerated and frozen yogurt and reduced-fat milk.
  - Black heads of household have a positive, statistically significant effect on the purchase of bulk ice cream, sherbet/ice milk, refrigerated and drinkable yogurts, whole and canned milk, and butter. Asian heads of household have a positive, statistically significant effect on the purchase of all fluid milks, refrigerated and drinkable yogurts, and bulk ice cream.
  - Households in the Western, Eastern, and Central regions of the United States are more likely to purchase refrigerated yogurt, natural cheese, cottage cheese, and butter than those in the Southern region. Households in the Western region are also more likely to purchase frozen and drinkable yogurts and sherbet/ice milk.
  - Of the income categories analyzed, households in the two lowest categories—$20,000-$34,999 annually and $19,999 or less—have a positive, statistically significant influence on whole and reduced-fat milk purchases. Other dairy product purchases that are statistically significant and positively influenced by households with incomes of $34,999 or less include sherbet/ice milk, processed and cottage cheese, and margarine.

How Was the Study Conducted?

The authors compiled data on retail purchases of dairy products from Nielsen Homescan data for 2007. The Nielsen Homescan data provide detailed information on dairy product purchases for at-home use by U.S. households, allowing the authors to examine consumption patterns among margarine and

12 categories of dairy products: bulk ice cream, sherbet/ice milk, refrigerated yogurt, frozen yogurt, drinkable yogurt, whole milk, reduced-fat milk, canned milk, natural cheese, processed cheese, cottage cheese, and butter. The Nielsen database includes not only economic data such as product prices, but also demographic and location information. The authors used the data to derive estimates of own- and cross-price elasticities and expenditure elasticities for the 13 product categories, employing a censored demand system.

INTRODUCTION

A wide array of milk and dairy products is offered by the U.S. dairy industry to consumers. Over the past two decades, dairy demand analyses have been conducted at the aggregated and disaggregated levels, using panel and cross-sectional data. Although several methods have been used to derive dairy demand parameter estimates, one of the most popular has been the Almost Ideal Demand System (AIDS) model and its many variations. (See, for example, Chouinard et al. (2010), Huang and Lin (2000), Maynard and Veeramani (2003), Maynard and Liu (1999), and Heien and Wessells (1990)).

In this study, a censored demand system used by Dong, Gould, and Kaiser (2004) is employed to estimate the demand for four major dairy categories: fluid milk, ice cream, yogurt, and cheese. These four broad categories are disaggregated into three fluid milks, two ice creams, three yogurts, and three cheeses, plus butter and margarine. The objective of the study is to estimate demand elasticities with respect to retail prices, expenditure, and several demographic variables.

BACKGROUND

While there are numerous studies focusing on aggregated dairy products, few display an analysis of the many disaggregated products for dairy goods available in retail stores. The authors make no effort to catalog the relevant earlier studies. One of the studies most comparable to the present analysis was conducted by Chouinard et al. (2010). Using weekly Information Resources Incorporated's (IRI) Infoscan[TM] scanner data for the years 1997 through 1999, Chouinard estimated price and income elasticities at the city level from an Incomplete Almost Ideal Demand System that is linear in income and linear and quadratic in prices. Findings showed that the own-price elasticities for 1-percent milk (–0.88), 2-percent milk (–0.79), no-fat or skim milk (–0.62), whole milk (–0.74), natural cheese (–0.72), processed cheese (–0.77), shredded cheese (–0.25), butter (–0.41), ice cream (–0.80), and flavored yogurt (–0.77) were smaller than the elasticities estimated by our censored demand system at the household level.

Maynard and Liu (1999) estimated three separate models, a quantity-dependent double-log specification, a linearized AIDS model, and a differential demand system model, using weekly national average retail scanner data from Nielsen (formerly referred to as A.C. Nielsen) for the years 1996 through 1998. Results from the linearized AIDS model, which is the model most similar to that used in the present study, revealed that own-price elasticities for flavored milk, shredded cheese, frozen yogurt, and frozen novelties were elastic. The estimates from the differential demand system also showed these dairy products to be elastic, but provided elastic results for butter and ice cream in addition.

In the two studies above, Chouinard et al. and Maynard and Liu avoided the data-censoring problem by aggregating the data from household to city or national level. Heien and Wessells (1990) applied the AIDS model to estimate a demand system that includes 11 food items, with a focus on dairy. In their study, a two-step censored regression approach was compared with an uncensored approach, using data retrieved from USDA's 1977-78 household food consumption survey (HFCS). Own-price elasticities for milk, cheese, cottage cheese, butter, margarine, and ice cream were all inelastic under the censored demand estimation, but were elastic for ice cream, cottage cheese, and butter. The uncensored demand model expenditure elasticities were lower for all items than they were for the censored demand model, ranging from 0.61 to 0.89.

A study by Boehm and Babb (1975) used two separate models without censoring to estimate price and expenditure elasticities at the market level for dairy products, using cross-sectional and time-series data from the United Dairy Industry Association. Findings from the model showed that national average own-price elasticities for whole milk (–1.70), 2% milk (–1.33), buttermilk (–1.52), cottage cheese (–1.29), processed cheese (–1.71), and canned milk (–1.33) were all elastic, while other dairy products such as ice cream (–0.42), ice milk (–0.56), American cheese (–0.44), butter (–0.76), and yogurt (–0.31) were less than 1 in magnitude. All of the expenditure elasticity estimates for the above dairy products were also less than 1.

A CENSORED DEMAND SYSTEM MODEL WITH ADDING-UP CONSTRAINT

The present study uses Nielsen 2007 Homescan data, which provide detailed dairy product purchases at the retail level for at-home use by U.S. households. Household demographic variables are also collected and combined with the purchase data. An analyst needs to address the data-censoring problem when using these household data, particularly for a system of demand analysis. Normally, not every product from the system will be purchased by any given household for the data survey period (1 year). Ignoring this nonpurchase issue could lead to biased parameter estimates (Wales and Woodland, 1983). To solve this censoring problem, we define the share equations as:

$$S^* = A + \gamma \ln P + \xi \ln Y + \varepsilon,$$
(1)

where S^* is a column vector of latent expenditure shares on M products. Equation 1, the AIDS model specified by Deaton and Muellbauer (1980), is derived from the price-independent generalized logarithmic (PIGLOG) utility function for a consumer. P is a column vector of the associated M product prices, and is the deflated total dairy expenditure, with y^* as total P expenditure and P^* as a translog price index. The ε is a column vector of M error terms.

In order to obtain the effects of household demographic variables on dairy demand, we incorporate these variables into the AIDS model through transformation of the intercept A of equation 1. We follow Abdulai (2002) by defining the intercept of equation 1 as:

$$A = \beta_0 + \beta X,$$
(2)

where X is a column vector of N demographic variables. The translog price index P^* is defined as:

$$\ln P^* = \alpha_0 + A' \ln P + \frac{1}{2}(\ln P)' \gamma (\ln P).$$
(3)

In equations 1, 2, and 3, β_0 (M x 1), β (M x N), γ (M x M), ξ (M x 1), and α_0 (a scalar) are parameters to be estimated.

The latent expenditure shares of equation 1 are derived from the utility maximization problem under the budget constraint, and they must sum to 1 (adding-up). The adding-up and other theoretical constraints, such as symmetry and homogeneity, are attained through parameter restrictions. However, no restriction is imposed to ensure that the latent shares S^* lie between 0 and 1. To account for this non-negativity and the adding-up of the observed shares S, Wales and Woodland (1983) developed a mapping rule, later used by Dong, Gould, and Kaiser (2004), which transforms the latent shares S^* to the observed shares S as:

$$
S_i = \begin{cases} \dfrac{S_i^*}{\sum\limits_{j \in \Delta} S_j^*}, & \text{if } S_i^* > 0, \\[2mm] 0, & \text{if } S_i^* \leq 0, \end{cases} \qquad (i = 1, 2, \cdots, M),
$$

(4)

where the subscript Δ is a set of all positive shares' subscripts. Equation 4 guarantees that the observed shares lie between 0 and 1 and sum to unity for each observation. Given equations 1 through 4, the likelihood function for this model can be derived for estimation.[1]

Elasticity Evaluation

Given the parameter estimates, demand elasticities of the latent system defined by equation 1 can be derived using the formula provided by Green and Alston (1990). Homogeneity and symmetry are held in these elasticities. Demand elasticities of the observed system defined by equation 4 can be obtained using a simulation procedure developed by Phaneuf, Kling, and Herriges (2000) and later applied by Dong, Gould, and Kaiser. Following Dong et al., assume R equals replicates of the M error term vectors ε in equation 1. The rth simulated latent share vector, , evaluated at the sample means of the exogenous variables (indicated by a bar over a variable), is:

$$
S_r^* = A + \gamma \ln \overline{P} + \xi \ln \frac{\overline{Y}}{P^*} + \varepsilon_r,
$$

(5)

where ε_r is the rth replicate of ε. The rth replicate of the ith observed share is:

$$
S_{ir} = \begin{cases} \dfrac{S_{ir}^*}{\sum\limits_{j \in \Delta} S_{jr}^*}, & \text{if } \ S_{ir}^* > 0, \\[4mm] 0, & \text{if } \ S_{ir}^* \le 0. \end{cases}
$$

(6)

The expected observed share vector for R replicates is calculated as a simple average of these simulated values:

$$
E(S) = \frac{1}{R} \sum_{r=1}^{R} S_r .
$$

(7)

If there is a small change in price j, ΔP_j, then the elasticity vector with respect to this price change is:

$$
\psi_j^Q = -\Lambda_j + \frac{\Delta E(S)}{\Delta E(P_j)} \cdot \frac{E(P_j) + \Delta E(P_j)/2}{E(S) + \Delta E(S)/2} ,
$$

(8)

where Λ_j is a vector of 0's with the jth element equal to 1, and $\Delta E(S)$ is the change in the simulated $E(S)$ given the change of expected price, $\Delta E(P_j)$. Homogeneity still holds in the elasticities of the observed system because the budget constraint (adding-up) is imposed in both latent and observed systems.

Most of the empirical estimations of price and expenditure elasticities reported in published analyses vary in size due to model specification. This study differs from other cross-sectional models in its ability to satisfy both non-negativity and the adding-up conditions. The Tobit system estimator (Amemiya, 1974) used by Yen, Lin, and Smallwood (2003) addressed the non-negativity, but the adding-up restriction is compromised. Other approaches, including the maximum entropy estimator of Golan, Perloff, and Shen (2001) (also a Tobit system), the sample-selection estimator (Yen and Lin, 2006), its two-step alternative (Shonkwiler and Yen, 1999), a semiparametric extension (Sam and Zheng, 2010), and other two-step estimators (Perali and Chavas, 2000; Meyerhoefer, Ranney, and Sahn, 2005; Heien and Wessells, 1990), also do not satisfy the adding-up constraint. The present study also differs in that it uses finer distinctions in the product categories selected—bulk ice cream, sherbet/ice milk, refrigerated yogurt, frozen yogurt, drinkable yogurt, whole milk, reduced-fat milk, canned milk, natural cheese, processed cheese, cottage cheese, butter, and margarine—to reduce potential aggregation biases in estimation.

Data

A demand system of 12 dairy products and margarine that were assumed separable from other food products is specified and estimated in this study. The impact of changes in retail prices, consumer expenditure, and demographic factors on these product purchases is determined. The data underlying the analysis are from Nielsen Homescan data for 2007. A sample of the U.S. population was used in the selection process of U.S. consumers who agreed to allow their grocery receipts of purchases made during a 12-month period to be scanned. Thirteen categories were established, using the descriptions of the UPC (United Product Code) and designated codes for each item. Individual overall quantities and expenditures are reported for all 13 products. Prices (unit values) are derived from observed quantities and expenditures after accounting for any coupons or promotions that might have been in effect. There are 63,061 households in this study, each of which purchased at least 1 of the 13 products in the 2007 data. The purchase record is matched to a household record that contains information on the size and composition of the household, income, age, race, gender, education and occupation of household members, and market location data. Projection factors (sample weights) are included in the Nielsen data to be used at the household level to provide estimates for the U.S. population. Although some researchers have heavily criticized the reliability of Nielsen data, the overall accuracy of self-reported data by Homescan panelists seems to be in line with many other surveys of this type (Einav, Leibtag, and Nevo, 2008).

Nielsen data contain only retail purchases for "at-home" use. Thus, one of the limitations of using the Nielsen data is that any of the 13 products consumed "away-from-home" at establishments such as fast food or dine-in restaurants, cafeterias, and schools are not included. If the products being analyzed have significant "away-from-home" purchases, estimated economic measures such as per capita consumption or elasticities must be evaluated with that in mind.

ESTIMATION RESULTS

Sample Statistics

According to Nielsen 2007 Homescan data, on average, consumers purchased more reduced-fat and whole milk than they did any other fluid-ounce dairy products (table 1). Among dry-ounce products, refrigerated yogurt is the one most purchased, followed by margarine and processed and natural cheese. Dairy expenditures are largest for reduced-fat milk and bulk ice cream, which account for almost 42 percent of total dairy expenditures. Natural cheese had the highest average price among the seven dry-ounce products, while drinkable yogurt had the highest average price among the six fluid-ounce products.

In addition to prices, quantities, and expenditure, demographic-variable summary statistics are also displayed in table 1. Variables used in the analysis include household size; age of female head of household and dummy variables representing children under the age of 6 years; teenagers 13-17 years; single (unmarried) head of household; White, Black, Asian, and Other (other race) heads of household; U.S. region (East, Central, Southern, and West); and female head educational attainment (up to some college), along with seven household income categories ranging from 0 to $150,000 or more per year.[2] To avoid singularity problems, the demographic dummy variables of Southern region, White head of household, and household income of $150,000 or more per year are used as the base.

Summary of Estimated Demand System Price and Demographic Coefficients

Tables 2 and 3 show the coefficient estimates derived from demand systems consisting of 13 different products and 18 demographic variables. A total of 338 parameters (among them 234 are demographics, 91 are prices, and 13 are total expenditures) were estimated using the GAUSS software system and BHHH maximum likelihood procedure (Berndt et al., 1974). Of the 234 demographic parameter estimates, 154 are statistically significant at the 10-percent level or better. All of the own-price coefficients are statistically different from zero at the 10-percent level of significance except for margarine. Of the 78 cross-price coefficients estimated, 58 (74 percent) were statistically significant at the 10-percent level or better. Eleven of the 13 estimated expenditure coefficients were statistically significant at the 10-percent level or better.

Table 1. Variable definitions and sample statistics (sample size = 63,061)

Variable	Mean	SD	% of households purchasing
	Quantities (oz or floz per household over 12 months)		
Bulk ice cream (floz)	591.77	801.69	89
Ice milk & sherbet (floz)	22.36	104.90	18
Refrigerated yogurt (oz)	316.61	505.48	80
Frozen yogurt (oz)	16.77	137.61	8
Drinkable yogurt (floz)	27.13	131.80	18
Whole milk (floz)	609.37	1,746.28	49
Reduced-fat milk (floz)	2,755.11	3,525.58	27
Canned milk (floz)	33.42	117.27	43
Natural cheese (oz)	121.90	173.63	86
Processed cheese (oz)	146.31	164.70	94
Cottage cheese (oz)	85.63	183.61	57
Butter (oz)	82.54	135.25	65
Margarine (oz)	153.80	196.64	74
	Expenditures (dollars spent per household over 12 months)		
Bulk ice cream	32.73	45.04	
Ice milk & sherbet	1.09	5.52	
Refrigerated yogurt	27.96	44.94	
Frozen yogurt	1.03	9.42	
Drinkable yogurt	3.34	15.80	
Whole milk	16.91	45.93	
Reduced-fat milk	70.56	84.68	
Canned milk	2.66	8.08	
Natural cheese	29.81	40.33	
Processed cheese	26.70	29.60	
Cottage cheese	9.61	20.63	
Butter	13.67	22.07	
Margarine	10.56	13.67	
	Prices (dollars spent per oz or floz over 12 months)		
Bulk ice cream ($/floz)	$0.06	$0.04	

Table 1. (Continued)

Variable	Mean	SD	
	Prices (dollars spent per oz or floz over 12 months)		
Ice milk & sherbet ($/floz)	0.05	0.01	
Refrigerated yogurt ($/oz)	0.09	0.03	
Frozen yogurt ($/oz)	0.09	0.03	
Drinkable yogurt ($/floz)	0.13	0.04	
Canned milk ($/floz)	0.09	0.02	
Natural cheese ($/oz)	0.27	0.08	
Processed cheese ($/oz)	0.20	0.07	
Cottage cheese ($/oz)	0.12	0.02	
Butter ($/oz)	0.18	0.06	
Margarine ($/oz)	0.08	0.04	
	Demographic variables		
Continuous variables:			
Household size - number of members	2.43	1.31	
Average age of female head of household	52.00	11.71	
Dummy variables (1 = yes, 0 = otherwise) – Percent of households:			
Children less than 6 years old	9%		
Teenagers 13 – 17 years old	13		
Single person household	24		
Eastern region	17		
Central region	27		
Southern region (base)	36		
Western region	20		
Female head of household w/some college	30		
White head of household (base)	84		
Black head of household	9		
Asian head of household	2		
Other head of household	5		
Household income ≤$19,999	11		
Household income $20,000-34,999	20		
Household income $35,000-49,999	19		
Household income $50,000-69,999	20		
Household income $70,000-99,999	18		
Household income $100,000-149,999	10		
Household income ≥$150,000 (base)	2		

Note: "floz" is fluid ounce and "oz" is dry ounce. Income is per year.
Source: Authors' calculations, using 2007 Nielsen Homescan data.

Table 2. Censored demand system parameter estimates for demographics

Variable	Intercept	Household size	Age of female head of household	Children ages 6 and younger
Bulk ice cream	0.039*	−0.005*	0.001	−0.024*
Sherbet/ice milk	−0.026*	0.001*	0.000	−0.002
Refrigerated yogurt	0.207*	−0.003	−0.001*	0.017*
Frozen yogurt	−0.017*	0.002	0.000	−0.003*
Drinkable yogurt	0.038*	−0.003*	0.000*	0.010*
Whole milk	0.335*	0.004*	−0.001*	0.076*
Reduced-fat milk	−0.379*	0.002	−0.001*	−0.035*
Canned milk	−0.023*	0.000*	0.001*	−0.001*
Natural cheese	0.367*	−0.005*	−0.001*	0.000
Processed cheese	0.311*	0.005*	−0.001*	−0.023*
Cottage cheese	−0.045*	0.003	0.001*	−0.004
Butter	0.106*	−0.003	0.001*	−0.006
Margarine	0.086*	0.003	0.001*	−0.006

Variable	Teenagers ages 13-17	Single person household	Female head of household w/ some college	Black head of household
Bulk ice cream	0.008	0.014*	−0.003	0.053*
Sherbet/ice milk	0.000	0.001	0.000	0.008*
Refrigerated yogurt	−0.006	0.024*	0.035*	0.012*
Frozen yogurt	−0.002*	0.005*	0.001*	0.000
Drinkable yogurt	−0.006*	0.005*	0.001	0.007*
Whole milk	−0.009	−0.025*	−0.035*	0.055*
Reduced-fat milk	0.032*	0.035*	0.020*	−0.093*
Canned milk	−0.001*	−0.006*	−0.001	0.020*
Natural cheese	−0.006	0.002	0.011*	−0.024*
Processed cheese	0.002	−0.017*	−0.015*	−0.025*
Cottage cheese	−0.008*	−0.003*	−0.001	−0.042*
Butter	−0.002*	−0.009*	−0.001	0.012*
Margarine	−0.001	0.025*	−0.013*	0.016

Variable	Asian head of household	Other-race head of household	Eastern region	Central region
Bulk ice cream	−0.002	0.000	−0.002*	0.001
Sherbet/ice milk	0.001	0.002	0.010*	−0.004

Table 2. (Continued)

Variable	Asian head of household	Other-race head of household	Eastern region	Central region
Refrigerated yogurt	0.043*	0.013*	0.037*	0.020*
Frozen yogurt	0.002	−0.002	0.002*	−0.003*
Drinkable yogurt	0.011*	0.005*	0.001	0.000*
Whole milk	0.042*	0.039*	−0.025*	−0.075*
Reduced-fat milk	0.026*	−0.025*	−0.049*	0.008*
Canned milk	0.011*	0.005*	−0.009*	−0.002*
Natural cheese	−0.056*	0.006	0.016*	0.012*
Processed cheese	−0.035*	−0.014*	−0.022*	−0.004*
Cottage cheese	−0.031*	−0.009*	0.008*	−0.033*
Butter	−0.008	−0.009*	0.047*	0.024*
Margarine	−0.030	−0.007	−0.006	0.001

Variable	Western region	Household income ≤$19,999	Household income $20,000–$34,999	Household income $35,000–$49,999
Bulk ice cream	0.003*	0.003	0.003	0.003*
Sherbet/ice milk	0.004*	0.001	−0.004	0.004
Refrigerated yogurt	0.037*	−0.073*	−0.060	−0.054*
Frozen yogurt	0.002	−0.008*	−0.006*	−0.005*
Drinkable yogurt	0.002	−0.006*	−0.011*	−0.009*
Whole milk	−0.054*	0.081*	0.053*	0.041*
Reduced-fat milk	−0.055*	0.002	0.013*	0.007
Canned milk	−0.004*	0.003	0.000	0.001
Natural cheese	0.056*	−0.024*	−0.011*	−0.005
Processed cheese	−0.040*	0.017*	0.019*	0.023*
Cottage cheese	0.031*	0.007	0.006	0.003
Butter	0.043*	−0.046*	−0.033*	−0.025*
Margarine	−0.015	0.047*	0.036*	0.028*

Variable	Household income $50,000–$69,999	Household income $70,000–$99,999	Household income $100,000–$149,999	
Bulk ice cream	−0.015*	−0.017*	−0.018*	
Sherbet/ice milk	0.002	0.001	0.001	
Refrigerated yogurt	−0.044*	−0.032*	−0.025*	
Frozen yogurt	−0.005*	−0.002	−0.003*	

Variable	Household income $50,000–$69,999	Household income $70,000–$99,999	Household income $100,000–$149,999	
Drinkable yogurt	−0.009*	−0.005*	−0.005*	
Whole milk	0.023*	0.007	0.003	
Reduced-fat milk	0.015*	0.016*	0.014*	
Canned milk	0.002	0.000	0.000	
Natural cheese	0.002	0.007*	0.011*	
Processed cheese	0.020*	0.019*	0.014*	
Cottage cheese	0.004*	0.000*	0.003	
Butter	−0.016*	−0.007	−0.001	
Margarine	0.020	0.012	0.005	

Note: Level of statistical signifi cance: * = 10% or better. Income is per year.
Source: Authors' calculations, using 2007 Nielsen Homescan data.

Table 3. Censored demand system parameter estimates for price and total expenditures

Variable	Bulk ice cream	Sherbet/ ice milk	Refrig. yogurt	Frozen yogurt	Drinkable yogurt
	Total expenditure				
	0.006*	−0.002*	0.003*	0.000	−0.002*
	Price coefficients				
Bulk ice cream	−0.025*				
Sherbet/ice milk	−0.003*	−0.007*			
Refrigerated yogurt	0.005*	−0.004*	−0.041*		
Frozen yogurt	0.002*	−0.001*	−0.010*	−0.013*	
Drinkable yogurt	0.002*	0.002*	0.001	−0.006*	−0.038*
Whole milk	0.008	0.004*	0.004	0.008*	0.001
Reduced-fat milk	−0.024*	0.001	0.031*	0.009*	0.016*
Canned milk	−0.001*	0.005*	0.002*	0.001	0.003*
Natural cheese	0.01 5*	0.002*	−0.001	0.003*	0.003*
Processed cheese	−0.015*	−0.001	0.011*	0.003*	0.006*
Cottage cheese	0.002*	0.004*	−0.012*	0.000	0.003*
Butter	0.017*	−0.001	−0.003	−0.001	0.001
Margarine	−0.017*	−0.001	0.017*	0.006*	0.007*

Table 3. (Continued)

Variable	Bulk ice cream	Sherbet/ ice milk	Refrig. yogurt	Frozen yogurt	Drinkable yogurt
	Total expenditure				
	−0.051*	0.065*	0.003*	0.010*	−0.024*
	Price coefficients				
Bulk ice cream					
Sherbet/ice milk					
Refrigerated yogurt					
Frozen yogurt					
Drinkable yogurt					
Whole milk	−0.179*				
Reduced-fat milk	0.118*	−0.261*			
Canned milk	0.011*	0.008*	−0.014*		
Natural cheese	0.035*	0.054*	0.001	−0.147*	
Processed cheese	−0.014*	0.016*	−0.007*	0.024*	−0.006*
Cottage cheese	0.028*	0.012*	0.005*	0.002	0.010*
Butter	0.015*	0.025*	−0.006*	0.003*	0.000
Margarine	−0.021*	−0.004	−0.007*	0.006	−0.026*

Variable	Cottage Cheese	Butter	Margarine		
	Total expenditure				
	0.010*	−0.001	−0.033*		
	Price coefficients				
Bulk ice cream					
Sherbet/ice milk					
Refrigerated yogurt					
Frozen yogurt					
Drinkable yogurt					
Whole milk					
Reduced-fat milk					
Canned milk					
Natural cheese					
Processed cheese					
Cottage cheese	−0.062*				
Butter	0.005*	−0.070*			
Margarine	0.004*	0.019*	0.0170		

Notes: Level of statistical significance: * = 10% or better.
Source: Authors' calculations using 2007 Nielsen Homescan data.

COMPENSATED DEMAND ELASTICITIES

Two sets of demand elasticities can be derived from the censored AIDS model estimates: compensated (Hicksian) and uncompensated (Marshallian). According to economic theory, changes in both price and income can influence demand. A compensated demand curve allows income to change to "compensate" for the price change, while an uncompensated demand curve does not.

The compensated price elasticities for the 13 products are presented in table 4. Each cell shows the price elasticity for a change in the price of the product identified at the top of the column. All own-price elasticities are negative and statistically significant at the 10-percent level. The cross-price relationships estimated in large demand systems provide information about how the purchase price of one product affects the demand for another product. Of the 156 compensated cross-price elasticity estimates shown in table 4, 145 (93 percent) are statistically significant at the 10-percent level.

Table 4. Estimated compensated price elasticities

Variable	Bulk ice cream	Sherbet/ ice milk	Refrig. yogurt	Frozen yogurt	Drinkable yogurt
Bulk ice cream	−0.77*	0.00*	0.12*	0.01*	0.01*
Sherbet/ice milk	0.05*	−1.21*	−0.02	−0.04*	0.06*
Refrigerated yogurt	0.16*	−0.01*	−1.08*	−0.05*	0.01
Frozen yogurt	0.17*	−0.02	−0.08*	−1.26*	−0.10*
Drinkable yogurt	0.18*	0.04*	0.13*	−0.11*	−1.72*
Whole milk	0.09*	0.01*	0.14*	0.03*	0.01*
Reduced-fat milk	0.09*	0.01*	0.17*	0.02*	0.04*
Canned milk	0.11*	0.12*	0.15*	0.03*	0.07*
Natural cheese	0.21*	0.02*	0.09*	0.02*	0.01*
Processed cheese	0.05*	0.00	0.17*	0.01*	0.03*
Cottage cheese	0.17*	0.05*	−0.04*	0.00	0.04*
Butter	0.34*	−0.01	0.07*	−0.01*	0.01
Margarine	0.09*	0.00	0.15*	0.01*	0.01*
Variable	Whole milk	Reduced -fat milk	Canned milk	Natural cheese	Processed cheese
Bulk ice cream	0.01	0.23*	0.01*	0.18*	0.05*
Sherbet/ice milk	0.17*	0.33*	0.16*	0.20*	0.10*
Refrigerated yogurt	0.06*	0.46*	0.02*	0.12*	0.16*
Frozen yogurt	0.22*	0.45*	0.03*	0.18*	0.16*

Table 4. (Continued)

Variable	Whole milk	Reduced-fat milk	Canned milk	Natural cheese	Processed cheese
Drinkable yogurt	0.11*	0.56*	0.06*	0.17*	0.23*
Whole milk	−1.65*	0.73*	0.04*	0.28*	0.10*
Reduced-fat milk	0.26*	−1.26*	0.04*	0.26*	0.12*
Canned milk	0.27*	0.55*	−1.31*	0.12*	−0.06*
Natural cheese	0.20*	0.60*	0.02*	−1.61*	0.23*
Processed cheese	0.02*	0.36*	−0.04*	0.26*	−0.89*
Cottage cheese	0.31*	0.49*	0.07*	0.14*	0.20*
Butter	0.23*	0.61*	−0.06*	0.16*	0.12*
Margarine	−0.01*	0.31*	−0.01*	0.15*	0.06*

Variable	Cottage Cheese	Butter	Margarine
Bulk ice cream	0.04*	0.13*	−0.01*
Sherbet/ice milk	0.17*	0.02	0.01
Refrigerated yogurt	−0.02*	0.05*	0.14*
Frozen yogurt	0.03*	0.04*	0.19*
Drinkable yogurt	0.09*	0.07*	0.19*
Whole milk	0.12*	0.11*	−0.02*
Reduced-fat milk	0.08*	0.13*	0.04*
Canned milk	0.14*	−0.09*	−0.11*
Natural cheese	0.05*	0.07*	0.09*
Processed cheese	0.07*	0.04*	−0.08*
Cottage cheese	−1.64*	0.10*	0.10*
Butter	0.07*	−1.81*	0.28*
Margarine	0.04*	0.11*	−0.90*

Notes: Level of statistical significance: * = 10% or better. Own-price elasticities are in boldface.

Source: Authors' calculations, using 2007 Nielsen Homescan data.

UNCOMPENSATED DEMAND ELASTICITIES

Table 5 presents the uncompensated price elasticity estimates for the 13 product categories purchased by consumers from retail stores. All own-price elasticities are negative, statistically significant at the 10-percent level, and are relatively similar in size to the compensated own-price elasticities presented above. Among the 156 cross-price elasticity estimates, 133 (85 percent) are statistically significant at the 10-percent level or better. Expenditure elasticities are also presented in table 5. All of the expenditure elasticities are statistically significant and positive.

Seven of the 13 product categories have expenditure elasticities that are 1 or greater.

Table 5. Estimated uncompensated price and total expenditure elasticities

Variable	Bulk ice cream	Sherbet/ ice milk	Refrig. yogurt	Frozen yogurt	Drinkable yogurt
Bulk ice cream	−0.91*	−0.01*	0.01*	0.00*	−0.00
Sherbet/ice milk	−0.08*	−1.21*	−0.12*	−0.05*	0.05*
Refrigerated yogurt	0.02*	−0.02*	−1.19*	−0.05*	−0.00
Frozen yogurt	0.03*	−0.03*	−0.19*	−1.26*	−0.11*
Drinkable yogurt	0.05*	0.04*	0.03	−0.11*	−1.73*
Whole milk	−0.02*	0.01*	0.06*	0.03*	0.00
Reduced-fat milk	−0.07*	0.00*	−0.05*	0.02*	0.02*
Canned milk	−0.04*	0.11*	0.03*	0.03*	0.06*
Natural cheese	0.07*	0.01*	−0.02*	0.01*	0.00
Processed cheese	−0.07*	−0.01*	0.08*	0.00	0.02*
Cottage cheese	0.02*	0.05*	−0.15*	0.00	0.03*
Butter	0.20*	−0.01*	−0.04*	−0.02*	0.00
Margarine	−0.04*	0.00*	0.05*	0.01*	0.00
Variable	Whole milk	Reduced -fat milk	Canned milk	Natural cheese	Processed cheese
Bulk ice cream	−0.06*	−0.05*	0.00*	0.06*	−0.07*
Sherbet/ice milk	0.10*	0.08*	0.15*	0.09*	−0.01
Refrigerated yogurt	−0.01	0.18*	0.01*	0.00	0.04*
Frozen yogurt	0.16*	0.17*	0.02*	0.06*	0.04*
Drinkable yogurt	0.04*	0.30*	0.05*	0.06*	0.11*
Whole milk	−1.70*	0.52*	0.03*	0.19*	0.01
Reduced-fat milk	0.19*	−1.57*	0.03*	0.12*	−0.02*
Canned milk	0.20*	0.26*	−1.32*	0.00	−0.19*
Natural cheese	0.32*	0.00	0.02	−1.73*	0.10*
Processed cheese	−0.04*	0.13*	−0.05*	0.16*	−0.99*
Cottage cheese	0.23*	0.19*	0.05*	0.01	0.07*
Butter	0.17*	0.34*	−0.07*	0.05	0.01
Margarine	−0.08*	0.05*	−0.02*	0.03*	−0.05*
Variable	Cottage Cheese	Butter	Margarine	Total expenditure	
Bulk ice cream	0.01*	0.07*	−0.06*	1.01*	
Sherbet/ice milk	0.13*	−0.04*	−0.04*	0.93*	
Refrigerated yogurt	−0.06*	−0.01	0.09*	1.00*	
Frozen yogurt	−0.01	−0.02*	0.14*	1.00*	

Table 5. (Continued)

Variable	Cottage Cheese	Butter	Margarine	Total expenditure	
Drinkable yogurt	0.06*	0.02	0.14*	0.96*	
Whole milk	0.10*	0.07*	−0.06*	0.77*	
Reduced-fat milk	0.04*	0.06*	−0.02*	1.14*	
Canned milk	0.11*	−0.15*	−0.17*	1.06*	
Natural cheese	0.01*	0.01*	0.03*	1.04*	
Processed cheese	0.04*	−0.01	−0.12*	0.85*	
Cottage cheese	**−1.68***	0.04*	0.05*	1.10*	
Butter	0.04*	**−1.87***	0.23*	0.97*	
Margarine	0.00	0.06*	**−0.95***	0.94*	

Note: Level of statistical significance: * = 10% or better. Own-price elasticities are in boldface.

Source: Authors' calculations, using 2007 Nielsen Homescan data.

ESTIMATED ELASTICITIES OF DEMOGRAPHIC VARIABLES

Table 6 displays the impact of demographic variables on the demand for "at-home" dairy products and margarine. Eighteen exogenous demographic variables are analyzed in the censored demand model, including household size, children under 6 years, teens age 13-17, average age of female heads of household, single person household, households living in the Eastern, Central, and Western regions of the United States, female heads of household who have some college training, Asian, Black, and Other race household heads, and six household income categories. Findings from the censored demand system show that the size of households is statistically significant and positively influences the purchase of sherbet/ice milk, drinkable yogurts, whole milk, reduced-fat milk, processed cheese, and margarine. Although there are more women in the workforce today than 20 years ago, women still do the majority of the shopping and cooking for the household (Babble, 2010; Casual Kitchen, 2010). Purchases of dairy items, including bulk ice cream, sherbet/ice milk, frozen yogurt, canned milk, cottage cheese, and butter, are all statistically significant and positively influenced by the age of the female head of household.

Table 6. Estimated demographic elasticities

Variable	Intercept	Household size	Age of female head of household	Children ages 6 and younger	Teenagers ages 13-17	Single-person household	Female head of household w/some college
Bulk ice cream	-0.295*	-0.037*	0.248*	-0.006	0.002*	0.012*	-0.007*
Sherbet/ice milk	-1.256*	0.115*	0.069*	-0.002	0.000	0.003	0.000
Refrigerated yogurt	0.503*	-0.024*	-0.229*	0.007*	-0.004*	0.027*	0.060*
Frozen yogurt	-0.822*	0.005	0.027*	-0.005*	-0.006*	0.021*	0.010*
Drinkable yogurt	0.193*	0.148*	-0.405*	0.015*	-0.013*	0.023*	0.008
Whole milk	0.976*	0.045*	-0.145*	0.027*	-0.005*	-0.032*	-0.062*
Reduced-fat milk	-1.339*	0.013*	-0.053*	-0.005	0.008*	0.020*	0.016*
Canned milk	-0.981*	0.019	0.594*	-0.001	-0.004*	-0.044*	-0.013*
Natural cheese	1.394*	-0.059*	-0.264*	0.001	-0.004*	0.000	0.018*
Processed cheese	1.289*	0.069*	-0.131*	-0.009*	0.000	-0.027*	-0.035*
Cottage cheese	-0.941*	-0.079*	0.436*	-0.003	-0.011*	-0.011*	-0.006
Butter	0.814*	-0.087	0.646*	-0.005*	-0.003*	-0.030*	-0.006*
Margarine	-0.158*	0.069*	-0.131*	-0.009	0.000	-0.027*	-0.035*

Variable	Black head of household	Asian head of household	Other race head of household	Eastern region	Central region	Western region	Household income ≤ $19,999
Bulk ice cream	0.022*	0.003*	0.000	0.001	-0.018*	-0.004*	0.001
Sherbet/ice milk	0.027*	-0.002	0.000	-0.010*	-0.005	0.015*	0.014*

Table 6. (Continued)

Variable	Black head of household	Asian head of household	Other race head of household	Eastern region	Central region	Western region	Household income ≤ $19,999
Refrigerated yogurt	0.007*	0.005*	0.003*	0.028*	0.023*	0.033*	-0.037*
Frozen yogurt	0.002	0.001	-0.002*	0.008*	-0.012*	0.007*	-0.018*
Drinkable yogurt	0.013*	0.005*	0.004*	0.002	0.003	0.010*	-0.012*
Whole milk	0.025*	0.004*	0.008*	-0.018*	-0.091*	-0.046*	0.043*
Reduced-fat milk	-0.019*	0.002*	-0.002*	-0.019*	0.002	-0.025*	0.002*
Canned milk	0.049*	0.006*	0.005*	-0.036*	-0.011*	-0.017	0.009
Natural cheese	-0.009*	-0.007*	0.002*	0.013*	0.014*	0.055*	-0.012*
Processed cheese	-0.011*	-0.005*	-0.003*	-0.019*	-0.007*	-0.041*	0.012*
Cottage cheese	-0.041*	-0.008*	-0.004*	0.016*	0.098*	0.069*	0.010*
Butter	0.015*	-0.003*	-0.004	0.093*	0.080*	0.101*	-0.062*
Margarine	-0.001*	-0.005*	-0.003	-0.019*	-0.007*	-0.041*	0.012*

Variable	Household income $20,000–$34,999	Household income $35,000–$49,999	Household income $50,000–$69,999	Household income $70,000–$99,999	Household income $100,000–$149,999		
Bulk ice cream	-0.006*	-0.007*	-0.011*	-0.012*	-0.007*		
Sherbet/ice milk	0.021*	0.022*	0.012	0.007	0.004		
Refrigerated yogurt	-0.054*	-0.047*	-0.038*	-0.026*	-0.011*		
Frozen yogurt	-0.023*	-0.016*	-0.017*	-0.008*	-0.006*		
Drinkable yogurt	-0.042*	-0.031*	-0.031*	-0.018*	-0.008*		

Variable	Household income $20,000–$34,999	Household income $35,000–$49,999	Household income $50,000–$69,999	Household income $70,000–$99,999	Household income $100,000–$149,999
Whole milk	0.050*	0.037*	0.021*	0.006	0.001
Reduced-fat milk	0.008*	0.004*	0.007*	0.007*	0.003*
Canned milk	0.003	0.005	0.010	0.000	0.000
Natural cheese	−0.010*	−0.003	0.002	0.006*	0.005*
Processed cheese	0.021*	−0.025*	0.021*	0.018*	0.007*
Cottage cheese	0.014*	0.007*	0.007*	0.000*	0.003*
Butter	−0.079*	−0.057*	−0.036*	−0.015	−0.001
Margarine	0.022*	0.025*	0.021*	0.018*	0.007

Note: Level of statistical significance: * = 10% or better. Income is per year.

Source: Authors' calculations, using 2007 Nielsen Homescan data.

Single-person heads of household, along with college-educated female heads of household, positively influenced the purchase of healthy dairy products such as refrigerated and frozen yogurt and reduced-fat milk. Black heads of household have a positive, statistically significant effect on purchases of bulk ice cream, sherbet/ice milk, refrigerated and drinkable yogurts, whole and canned milk, and butter. Asian heads of household also have a positive, statistically significant effect on purchases of bulk ice cream, refrigerated and drinkable yogurts, and all fluid milks. Households residing in the Eastern, Central, and Western regions of the United States have a greater impact on refrigerated yogurt, natural and cottage cheese, and butter than other dairy products and margarine. Of the income categories analyzed, households in the two lowest categories—$20,000-$34,999 annually and $19,999 or less—have a positive, statistically significant influence on purchases of whole and reduced-fat milk. Other dairy products that are statistically significant and positively influenced by households who make $34,999 or less include purchases of sherbet/ice milk, processed and cottage cheese, and margarine. Although the influence of most demographic variables is relatively small, some of them do have statistically significant effects on consumer purchases of dairy products.

CONCLUSION

This research estimated demand elasticities that can be used for policy analysis by researchers in academic institutions and policy-oriented agencies. An empirical analysis of Nielsen 2007 Homescan retail purchase data was used to estimate a censored demand system of margarine and 12 dairy products. Results indicate that dairy purchases are influenced by price, overall dairy expenditure, and demographic factors. Ten of the 12 uncompensated own- price elasticities for dairy products are statistically significant and elastic with respect to changes in retail prices. Similar findings are noted for compensated own-price elasticities.

Other findings reveal that consumers' purchases of bulk ice cream, refrigerated and frozen yogurts, reduced-fat milk, canned milk, natural cheese, and cottage cheese are sensitive to changes in overall dairy expenditures. Strong substitution relationships are found among bulk ice cream, reduced-fat milk, and natural cheese and other products in the demand system. The three fluid milks—whole milk, reduced-fat milk, and canned milk— are found to be strong substitutes for each other. Similar substitution relaionships exist among the three cheese products, natural cheese, cottage cheese, and processed cheese.

REFERENCES

Abdulai, A. (2002). "Household Demand for Food in Switzerland: A Quadratic Almost Ideal Demand System," *Swiss Journal of Economics and Statistics 138*, 1-18.

Amemiya, T. (1974). "Multivariate Regression and Simultaneous Equation Models when the Dependent Variables are Truncated Normal," *Econometrica 42*, 999-1012.

Babble for a new generation of parents (2010). http://www.babble.com/ CS/blogs/homework/archive/2010/03/17/working-moms-we-may-not-quot-doit-all-quot-anymore-but-we-still-quot-do-most-of-it-quot.aspx. Accessed on October 13, 2010.

Berndt, E., Hall, B. Hall, R. & Hausman, J. (1974). "Estimation and Inference in Nonlinear Structural Models," *Annals of Economic and Social Measurement 3*, 653-65.

Boehm, W. T. & Babb, E. M. (1975). "*Household Consumption of Beverage Milk Products.*" Station Bulletin 75. Department of Agricultural Economics, Agricultural Experiment Station, Purdue University, West Lafayette, IN.

Casual Kitchen (2010). "*Who Does the Cooking In Your Home? The Results May Surprise You.*" http://casualkitchen.blogspot.com/2010/08/ who-doescooking-in-your-home-results.html. Accessed on October 13, 2010.

Chouinard, H. H., LaFrance, J. T., Davis, D. E. & Perloff, J. M. (2010). "Milk Marketing Order Winners and Losers," *Applied Economic Review Perspective and Policy, 32*, 59-76.

Deaton, A. & Muellbauer, J. (1980). "An Almost Ideal Demand System," *American Economic Review, 70*, 312-36.

Dong, D., Gould, B. W. & Kaiser, H. (2004). "Food Demand in Mexico: An Application of the Amemiya-Tobin Approach to the Estimation of a Censored Food System," *American Journal of Agricultural Economics, 86*, 1094-1107.

Einav, L., Leibtag, E. & Nevo, A. (2008). *On the Accuracy of Nielsen Homescan Data.* U.S. Dept. of Agriculture, Economic Research Service, ERR- 69, December. http://www.ers.usda.gov/Publications/ERR69/

Golan, A., Perloff, J. M. & Shen, E. Z. (2001). "Estimating a Demand System with Non-negativity Constraints: Mexican Meat Demand," *The Review of Economics and Statistics, 83*, 541–50.

Gould, B. W., Cox, T. L. & Perali, F. (1991). "Demand for Food Fats and Oils: The Role of Demographic Variables and Government Donations," *American Journal of Agricultural Economics, 73*, 212-21.

Green, R. & Alston, J. M. (1990). "Elasticities in AIDS models," *American Journal of Agricultural Economics, 72*, 442-45.

Heien, D. & Wessells, C. R. (1990). "Demand Systems Estimation with Microdata: A Censored Regression Approach," *Journal of Business and Economic Statistics, 8*, 365-371.

Huang, K. S. & Lin, B. (2000). *Estimation of Food Demand and Nutrient Elasticities from Household Survey Data.* U.S. Dept. of Agriculture, Economic Research Service, Technical Bulletin 1887. August. http://www.ers.usda.gov/publications/tb1887/tb1887.pdf

Maynard, L. J. & Liu, D. (1999). *"Fragility in Dairy Product Demand Analysis."* Selected paper presentation at the annual meeting of the American Agricultural Economics Association, Nashville, TN, August 8-11.

Maynard, J. L & Veeramani, V. N. (2003). "Price Sensitivities for U.S. Frozen Dairy Products," *Journal of Agricultural and Applied Economics, 35*, 599-609.

Meyerhoefer, C. D., Ranney, C. K. & Sahn, D. E. (2005). "Consistent Estimation of Censored Demand Systems Using Panel Data," *American Journal of Agricultural Economics, 87*, 660–72.

Perali, F. & Chavas, J. P. (2000). "Estimation of Censored Demand Equations from Large Cross-Section Data," *American Journal of Agricultural Economics, 82*, 1022–37.

Phaneuf, D.J., Kling, C. L. & Herriges, J. A. (2000). "Estimation and Welfare Calculations in a Generalized Corner Solution Model with an Application to Recreation Demand," *Review of Economics and Statistics, 82*, 83-92.

Sam, A. G. & Zheng, Y. (2010). "Semiparametric Estimation of Consumer Demand Systems with Micro Data," *American Journal of Agricultural Economics, 92*, 246–57.

Shonkwiler, J. S. & Yen, S. T. (1999). "Two-Step Estimation of a Censored System of Equations," *American Journal of Agricultural Economics, 81*, 972–82.

Wales, T. J. & Woodland, A. D. (1983). "Estimation of Consumer Demand Systems with Binding Non-Negativity Constraints," *Journal of Econometrics, 21*, 263-85.

Yen, S. T., Lin, B. & Smallwood, D. M. (2003). "Quasi and Simulated Likelihood Approaches to Censored Demand Systems: Food Consumption by Food Stamp Recipients in the United States," *American Journal of Agricultural Economics, 85*, 458-78.

Yen, S. T. & Lin, B. (2006). "A Sample Selection Approach to Censored Demand Systems," *American Journal of Agricultural Economics, 88*, 742–49.

End Notes

[1] For more details, refer to Dong, Gould, and Kaiser for the derivation of the likelihood function and the model estimation

[2] Female head indicates the mother of the household. If no female head is present in the household, the head will be used as a substitute.

In: Milk Consumption
Editor: Francisco Paul Buren

ISBN: 978-1-62948-008-4
© 2013 Nova Science Publishers, Inc.

Chapter 4

RETAIL AND CONSUMER ASPECTS OF THE ORGANIC MILK MARKET*

Carolyn Dimitri and Kathryn M. Venezia

ABSTRACT

Consumer interest in organic milk has burgeoned, resulting in rapid growth in retail sales of organic milk. New analysis of scanner data from 2004 finds that most purchasers of organic milk are White, high income, and well educated. The data indicate that organic milk carries the USDA organic seal about 60 percent of the time, most organic milk is sold in supermarkets, organic price premiums are large and vary by region, and most organic milk is branded.

INTRODUCTION

U.S. retail sales of organic milk have been growing since the mid-1990s, with sales of organic milk and cream edging over $1 billion in 2005, up 25 percent from 2004. At the same time, overall sales of milk have remained constant since the mid-1980s (Miller and Blayney, 2006), and organic milk and cream now make up an estimated 6 percent of retail milk sales.[1] The boost

---

* This is an edited, reformatted and augmented edition of a United States Department of Agriculture publication, Report LDP-M-155-01, dated May 2007.

in organic milk sales is part of a wider growing interest in organic products, which resulted in an average annual growth rate of retail sales of organic food of nearly 18 percent between 1998 and 2005. Rising consumer interest in organic milk has been accompanied by a newfound widespread availability of the product, and organic milk is now available in nearly all food retail venues, including conventional supermarkets and big-box stores, such as Costco or Wal-Mart (see box, "Retail Venues"). USDA implemented national organic standards and an accompanying organic logo in October 2002, clearing the way for further growth in the sector under one Federal production and handling rule. The USDA organic standards specify the production process for processing, distributing, and growing organic food, while the logo provides an easy way for consumers to recognize organic products (see box, "National Organic Standards"). The regulations were implemented in part to provide consumers with confidence that organic products have consistent, uniform standards (USDA, 2002b). Media reports indicate that supermarkets experienced significant shortages of organic milk during 2005 and 2006 (Oliver, 2006; Weinraub and Nicholls, 2005), suggesting that consumer demand is unmet at current market prices. Wal-Mart's announcement in 2006 of its intention to increase its offerings of organic food is likely to introduce new pressures in the organic dairy sector, which is already struggling to meet market demands. As of May 2007, two main suppliers provide approximately 75 percent of the Nation's branded organic milk: Organic Valley, an independent cooperative in business since 1988; and Horizon Organic, which has produced organic milk since 1992. Horizon merged with a conventional agribusiness firm in 2004. In 2003, independent firm Aurora Dairy entered the sector and began operating as a processor of private-label organic milk. As a result of this venture, by 2006, many major conventional supermarket chains had introduced private-label organic milk. Anecdotal evidence suggests that the three main organic dairies (of branded and private-label milk) are actively working to increase the supply of organic milk by recruiting and assisting conventional milk producers with the transition to organic production.[2]

To date, most characterizations of consumers who purchase organic products result from industry studies and offer conflicting views. The studies have focused on consumers of organic foods in general, not just consumers of organic milk. These market analyses use consumer surveys to gather information and have focused on trends in consumer purchases of organic foods (Whole Foods Market, 2005) and demographic characteristics of organic consumers (Hartman Group, 2004, 2002, 2000). The Whole Foods 2005 survey indicates that 65 percent of consumers have tried organic foods, 27 percent bought more organic food in 2005 than in 2004, and 10 percent consume organic food several times a week. The most recent Hartman study (2006) develops two indicators: an ethnic purchase index and a core consumer purchase index. The ethnicity analysis indicates that Asians and Hispanics are the ethnic groups (when considering Asians, Hispanics, Whites, and Blacks) most likely to have purchased organic products in the previous 3 months. The core consumer index, however, indicates that core consumers (defined by the Hartman Group as consumers committed to an organic lifestyle) are most likely to be Hispanic and Black (Baxter, 2006.) Earlier consumer surveys (administered in 2004 by the Hartman group) found that half of those who frequently buy organic food have incomes below $50,000 per year, and that Blacks, Asians and Hispanics use more organic products than the general population (Howie, 2004.) In 2004, 42 percent of organic consumers had annual incomes below $40,000 (Barry, 2004.)

RETAIL VENUES

Natural products channel—Consists of natural products supermarket chains, independent stores, and health food stores. Natural food supermarkets offer less-processed foods and more foods free of preservatives, hormones, and artificial ingredients.

Conventional supermarket—A format offering a full line of groceries, meat, and produce with at least $2 million in annual sales. These stores typically carry approximately 15,000 items and frequently offer a service deli and a bakery.

Superstore—A larger version of the conventional supermarket with at least 40,000 square feet in total selling area and 25,000 items. Superstores offer an expanded selection of nonfood items, including health and beauty products and general merchandise.

Supercenters—A large food-drug combination store and mass merchandiser under a single roof. Supercenters offer a wide variety of food, as well as nonfood merchandise, average more than 170,000 square feet, and typically devote as much as 40 percent of their space to grocery items.

Wholesale club—A membership retail/wholesale hybrid with a limited variety of products presented in a warehouse-type environment. These 120,000-squarefoot stores usually have 30 to 40 percent grocery sales and sell mostly large sizes and bulk sales.

Mass merchandiser—A store that primarily sells household items, electronic goods, and apparel but also offers packaged food products.

In contrast to the Hartman 2006 and 2004 results, earlier studies characterize organic consumers as White, affluent, well-educated, and concerned about health and product quality (Lohr, 2001; Richter et al., 2000; ITC, 1999; Thompson, 1998). These studies also cluster the average age of organic consumers in two age groups: 18-29 years and 45-49 years (Thompson, 1998; Lohr and Semali, 2000). One element that has remained generally accepted through the years is that parents of young children or infants are more likely than those without children to purchase organic food.

NATIONAL ORGANIC STANDARDS

Organic production relies on ecologically based practices, such as biological pest management and composting, and crops are produced on land that has had no prohibited substances applied to it for at least 3 years prior to harvest. Soil fertility and crop nutrients are managed through tillage and cultivation practices, crop rotations, and cover crops, supplemented with manure and crop waste material and allowed synthetic substances. Crop pests, weeds, and diseases are controlled through physical, mechanical, and biological control management methods. Organic farming systems virtually exclude the use of synthetic chemicals, antibiotics, and hormones in crop production; and prohibit the use of antibiotics and hormones in livestock production. Organic food cannot be produced using genetic engineering and other excluded methods, sewage sludge, or ionizing radiation.

Standards for handlers require that organic and conventionally grown ingredients be kept separate, and that organic ingredients be stored in containers that do not compromise the organic nature of the food. Both organic and conventional ingredients must not be treated with ionizing radiation, excluded methods, and synthetic solvents. When being stored and shipped, organic products cannot be shipped or packed in containers containing synthetic fungicide, preservative, or fumigant.

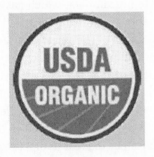

USDA implemented national organic standards in October 2002. These regulations require that organic growers and handlers (including food processors and distributors) be certified by a State or private agency accredited under the uniform standards developed by USDA, unless the farmers or handlers sell less than $5,000 a year in organic agricultural products. Retail food establishments that sell organically produced agricultural products but do not process them are also exempt from certification.

The national organic standards address the methods, practices, and substances used in producing and handling crops, livestock, and processed agricultural products. Although specific practices and materials used by organic operations may vary, the standards require every aspect of organic production and handling to comply with the provisions of the Organic Foods Production Act (OFPA). These standards include a national list of approved synthetic and prohibited nonsynthetic substances for use in organic production and handling. USDA organic standards for food handlers require that all nonagricultural ingredients, whether synthetic or nonsynthetic, be included on the national list.

Along with the national organic standards, USDA has strict labeling rules to help consumers know the exact organic content of the food they buy. The USDA organic seal also tells consumers that a product is at least 95 percent organic; use of the seal is voluntary, so not all foods with at least 95 percent organic ingredients will display the logo.

For further information, visit USDA's Agricultural Marketing Service/National Organic Program website at www.ams.usda.gov/nop/.

Consumer surveys provide insight into consumer behavior, and to date, most of the information and research on the organic industry is based on surveys. However, more reliable information about preferences can be obtained by examining scanner data on actual consumer purchases. This chapter relies on Nielsen Homescan data, which has demographic information and food purchase information for a national panel of households (see box, "Nielsen Homescan Panel Data"). The analysis uses data from 2004, which includes 38,375 households that purchased milk.

Organic milk is the focus of this analysis for two main reasons. First, the shortages of organic milk at the retail level are notable. Second, dairy— along with fresh produce and soymilk—is one of the first organic products consumers try; thus, it is likely to be purchased by a wide variety of people and may indicate future consumer interest in other organic products (Demeritt, 2004).

NIELSEN HOMESCAN PANEL DATA

This chapter uses the Nielsen Homescan panel, a nationwide panel of households that scanned their food purchases (from all retail outlets) at home. Data included detailed product characteristics, quantity, and expenditures for each food item purchased by each household. The data are unique in that they include detailed purchase information as well as demographic information about the households in the panel.

We used the full panel of 41,000 households. Households in the subset scanned only fixed-weight products (products with a universal product code, or UPC). From this set, we drew data from households that bought milk during 2004—38,375 households. Our sample is projectable to the U.S. universe of product purchases.

The data set is a stratified random sample. The sample was selected based on both demographic and geographic targets. Stratification was done to ensure that the sample matches the U.S. Census. The household was the primary sampling unit, and there was no intentional clustering. The weight assigned to each household reflects the demographic distribution within strata. All analysis relies on both the projection factor and strata to estimate proportions, means, and standard errors.

The analysis is conducted on a household level, where we aggregated purchase information for each household for 2004. We also created a new category "head of household," using the notion that most food shopping is done by women, making use of the demographic information Nielsen reports for both the female and male head of the household.

We used the information about educational level, age, and race/ethnicity for the female as the head of household except for the households without a female head. In that case, we used the information for the male. We also reclassified income; Nielsen reports income in categories, which we recalculated into four categories: "low" contains households with income of $24,999 or less; "middle" has households with incomes above $24,999 and less than or equal to $44,999; "upper" has income above $44,999 and less than or equal to $69,999; "high" is for income greater than $70,000.

RETAILING ORGANIC MILK HAS MANY DIMENSIONS

Retailing of organic milk has changed since the early 1990s, when most organic food was sold in specialty shops. Since then, organic food products have become available in a wide range of venues, with trends in retailing organic milk following those of conventionally produced food, including a growing reliance on private-label products. Two other features are unique aspects of retailing organic milk and other organic products: the USDA organic logo and price premiums. Marketing organic products is facilitated through the use of the USDA organic standards, which establish rules for the use of the label "organic" and the accompanying logo (see box, "National Organic Standards" on page 4). Organic milk, like most organic products, receives a price premium over conventional products.

Distribution Channels Differ for Organic and Conventional Milk

The wide availability of organic food in 2005[3] is in marked contrast to 1991, when 68 percent of organic food was sold in natural foods stores and 7 percent was sold through conventional channels, such as grocery stores, mass merchandisers, and club stores (table 1). In 2005, the share of organic food sold in natural foods stores had decreased to 48 percent, while the share sold through conventional channels increased to 46 percent. Conventional channels now sell the majority of organic milk, half and half, and cream products (76 percent) (Budgar, 2006).

Data on organic and conventional milk purchases by distribution channel indicate that nearly all organic milk is purchased in grocery stores (table 2), with about 9 percent of sales attributed to the natural products channel, which is defined here as the two major national natural products chains (Whole Foods and Wild Oats) and health food stores.[4] In contrast, conventional milk is purchased in a wider variety of venues, with 75 percent purchased in grocery stores, 10 percent purchased in supercenters, and 4 percent in club stores.

Private Label Used Less Often for Organic Milk, and Brand Names More Common

Private labeling for milk occurs at a much lower rate in the organic sector than in the conventional sector. In 2003, approximately 8 percent of all organic foods were sold under a private label (NBJ, 2004); in comparison, 16 percent of all food products were sold under a private label in the United States (ACNielsen, 2005). By 2005 (for the 12-month period ending the first quarter of 2005), it was estimated that the share of sales of private label organic products sales had risen to 16 percent in the United States (ACNielsen, 2005). The Nielsen Homescan data indicate that private-label organic milk made up 10 percent of organic milk purchases in 2004, while the two major brands of organic milk made up 80 percent. The two major brands—Organic Valley and Horizon Organic—belong to the first two companies to produce and distribute organic milk on a large scale. In contrast, private labeling of conventional milk dominates the dairy case, accounting for 64 percent of purchases. The conventional sector includes over 100 brands of milk, with no individual brand capturing more than approximately 1 percent of the market. With the entrance of Aurora Dairy into the organic milk market, and the consequent growth in private-label organic milk sold in conventional supermarkets, the share of sales of organic milk attributed to branded products may decrease in the coming years. In 2004, ERS calculations of the Nielsen Homescan data indicate that the national average price of conventional private-label milk was $1.88 per half gallon, compared with $3.65 for organic private-label milk, a price premium of $1.77. The organic price premiums for branded and private-label milk were similar, at 98 percent of the conventional price for branded and 94 percent for private label.

Table 1. Distribution of Organic Food Sales by Channel, 2005 and 1991

Channel	Organic sales, 2005	Share of total organic sales, 2005	Share of total organic sales, 1991
	$ millions	Percent	
Natural foods independent store	3,274	24	68
Natural foods grocery chain	3,253	24	NA
Conventional grocery	4,935	36	7
Mass merchandiser	689	5	NA
Club store	638	5	NA
Other	101	1	25
Farmers' market	486	4	NA
Food service	453	3	NA

Note: In 1991, farmers' market is included in the "other" category. NA = not available.
Source: Calculated by USDA, ERS from OTA, 2006.

Table 2. Percent of Milk Purchases and Average Retail Prices by Channel, 2004

Type of store	Organic milk		Conventional milk		Organic price premium
	Share of all sales	Average price	Share of all sales	Average price	
	Percent	Dollars	Percent	Dollars	Percent
Grocery stores	87	3.98	75	2.06	93
Drug stores	0	NA	3	1.83	NA
Mass merchandisers	0	3.63	2	1.80	101
Supercenters	7	4.08	10	1.84	122
Club stores	0	2.20	4	1.99	10
Other	5	4.98	3	2.19	127

Notes: The Nielsen dataset does not identify the natural products channel, which consists of natural products supermarkets (both chains and independents) and health food stores; thus, the grocery channel includes both conventional and natural products supermarkets and the "other" category includes health food stores and small independent stores. Percents do not sum to 100 because of rounding. Milk prices per half gallon were calculated by first calculating the average price per fluid ounce based on all sizes of milk purchased and multiplying this average by 64 ounces. NA = not available.
Source: Calculated by USDA, ERS from Nielsen data, using the Nielsen projection factor to weight the sample.

USDA Organic Logo Used More Often in Conventional Channels

Organic products may either display the word "organic" on the label or use the USDA organic logo, but in either case, the product has to satisfy the USDA requirements for use of the label organic (see box, "National Organic Standards" on page 4 for more information). Over time, consumers are gaining greater awareness of the USDA logo. In 2005, 40 percent of U.S. consumers noticed the logo, up from only 19 percent in 2003 (Whole Foods, 2005). In 2005, about 60 percent of organic food manufacturers displayed the USDA logo on their products, and over half of those who did not currently use the logo planned to use it in the future (OTA, 2006).

The Nielsen data reveal that the USDA organic logo was used on 54 percent of organic milk purchases in 2004 (table 3). The logo was used in conventional channels more often than in natural product channels. The difference in usage may arise because consumers who shop in natural products stores are more aware of organic food than consumers who shop in conventional supermarkets, and, thus, less reliant on the USDA organic logo to provide information about organic food. In conventional channels, 56 percent of organic milk purchases displayed the USDA organic logo, while just 39 percent of organic milk purchases carried the logo in the natural products channels. Private-label organic milk sported the USDA organic logo 51 percent of the time, while the top two brands of organic milk displayed the USDA organic logo 54 percent of the time. The usage of the organic label has most likely increased since 2004; after the implementation of the organic standards in October 2002, organic firms were given 18 months to revise package labels.

Organic Prices and Price Premiums Vary by Region

Prices of both organic and conventional milk vary by channel (see table 2), as does the price premium. Organic milk, like most organic products, receives a premium over conventional products. Organic consumers perceive that organic food provides environmental and health benefits, and thus are willing to pay a higher price (Onozaka et al., 2006).

Table 3. Use of USDA organic seal by major channels, 2004

Type of store	Organic milk purchases	
	USDA organic logo	Organic label only
	Percent	
Grocery stores	56	44
Supercenters	38	62
Other	36	64
Natural products	39	61
Total across all channels	54	46

Note: Organic labeled milk does not have the USDA organic logo but displays the word *organic* on the label and satisfies USDA regulations for use of the word *organic*. The stores in the natural products channel are also included in "grocery stores" and "other" (health food stores).
Source: Calculated by USDA, ERS from Nielsen data, using the Nielsen projection factor.

Price premiums persist over time when demand grows faster than supply; in the organic milk sector, demand for organic milk has been growing faster than supply since at least 2004. In 2004, the price premium for organic milk ranged from 10 percent to 127 percent of the conventional price. Most of the price premiums were closer to 100 percent, with only the few sales of organic milk in club stores receiving the 10-percent premium.

Table 4. Organic and conventional milk prices and organic premium by region, 2004

Region	Milk price per half gallon		Organic premium	
	Organic	Conventional		
	Dollars		*Dollars*	*Percent*
East	4.52	2.01	2.52	126
Central	3.81	1.85	1.96	106
South	2.80	2.01	1.79	89
West	3.90	2.27	1.63	72
National average	4.01	2.02	1.99	98

Note: Conventional and organic prices are averages of individual household purchases as reflected in the Nielsen Homescan data, using the Nielsen projection factor to appropriately weight the sample; price premiums and average prices are calculated by ERS. Price premiums in dollar terms are the difference between the price for organic and conventional milk; price premiums in percentage terms equal the premium divided by the conventional price.
Source: Calculated by USDA, ERS from Nielsen data, using the Nielsen projection factor.

Analysis of the Nielsen data indicates that milk prices vary by U.S. region. For conventional milk, the lowest average price per half gallon[5] is in the Central region ($1.85) and the highest is in the West ($2.27) (table 4); this regional variation in retail milk prices is consistent with previous work (see Leibtag, 2005). The lowest average price for organic milk is in the South ($2.80), and the highest is in the East ($4.52), with the national average price totaling $4.01. The price premium that organic milk commands over conventional milk is lowest in the West, at $1.63, or 72 percent of the conventional price. The organic premium is highest in the East, at $2.52, or 126 percent of the conventional price. The national average price premium for organic milk is $1.99, or 98 percent of the conventional price. Given that U.S. supermarkets are out of stock for organic milk from time to time, the high organic price premiums are not surprising (Weinraub and Nicholls, 2005; Oliver, 2006).

CHARACTERISTICS OF ORGANIC MILK HOUSEHOLDS

During 2004, 38,375 of the 41,000 households in the Nielsen panel purchased milk; 4 percent, or 1,489 of these households, purchased organic milk. Of these households, 45 percent spent less than 10 percent of their milk budget on organic milk; 17 percent spent between 10 and 30 percent on organic milk; 10 percent spent between 31 and 50 percent; 25 percent spent between 51 and 99 percent; and 4 percent bought only organic milk. In this analysis, the households that purchased some organic milk are referred to as "organic households" while the households that never purchased organic milk are "conventional households." The organic household category does not take into account systematic differences between frequent and infrequent buyers of organic milk.

Several demographic characteristics were found to be associated with the distribution of organic milk households relative to the distribution of conventional milk households, such as region, household income, education, and age of the head of household. Other factors, such as presence of children under 18 in the household and household size, had little relationship with the relative distribution of the two groups of consumers.

The distribution of organic households and of conventional households by demographic characteristics as shown in figures 1-6 is calculated by dividing the number of organic (or conventional) households in each region by the total number of organic (or conventional) households in the sample. This information is useful in that it provides insight into the characteristics that differentiate the typical organic household from the typical conventional household, plus it allows for a comparison of these results with those published by industry groups.

The data indicate that the share of organic households in the East and West exceeds each region's share of conventional milk households, while the opposite is true in the Central and South regions (figure 1). This finding may reflect the fact that consumers in the East and West have had access to organic food for a longer period of time, since natural products supermarkets (initially the major purveyor of organic food) have operated on the two coasts since the early 1990s and are just now moving into the Central and Southern regions. Distribution data by the age of households suggest that households headed by someone age 54 and younger are more likely to purchase organic milk (figure 2).

Household income and education of the head of the household seem to be associated with the likelihood that a household will buy organic or conventional milk. The data indicate that the share of organic households across income categories rises as income increases, and the high-income group is the only category where the proportion of households purchasing organic milk exceeds the proportion purchasing conventional milk (figure 3). Most (80 percent) organic milk consumers have at least attended some college, and those who have graduated from college or completed some post-graduate education make up 51 percent of organic milk consumers. The share of organic households with the highest two levels of education (graduated from college or completed some post-graduate studies) is greater than the share of conventional households with the same level of education (figure 4). What accounts for the association between income and education and purchasing organic milk? Household income and education are correlated, so income could be the factor driving the association with purchasing organic milk. Alternatively, education could be the driving factor, in that greater education may enhance one's understanding of the relationship between organic production techniques and environmental impacts.[6]

Reasonable explanations are lacking as to the association (or lack thereof) between some demographic factors and the distribution of organic milk households. For example, it is not clear why the share of organic households is less than the share of conventional households for Black and White households (figure 5). Similarly, while one might expect that larger households would buy much less organic milk than smaller households, particularly since smaller households have greater disposable income, household size appears to have little relationship with the propensity to purchase organic milk (figure 6).

In sum, the demographic data indicate that organic households are most likely to live in the West or East, be headed by someone age 54 or younger, have a college degree, and have annual household incomes of at least $70,000. They are less likely than conventional households to be Black. Conventional households are more likely to live in the South or Central regions, have annual household income less than $70,000, have not graduated from college, and be headed by a household head age 55 or older. Household size has little bearing on whether a household purchases only conventional milk, and the presence of children under age 18 has no bearing on the likelihood of a household to purchase organic or conventional milk.

Possible explanations for this characterization of the organic household is that "region" captures some other aspect that impacts the decision to buy organic milk, either an economic factor, such as price, or a noneconomic factor, such as interest in environmental issues. The importance of other factors—high income and a college degree—together suggest that organic households have higher discretionary income than conventional households and, thus, are able to afford and are willing to purchase higher priced organic milk.

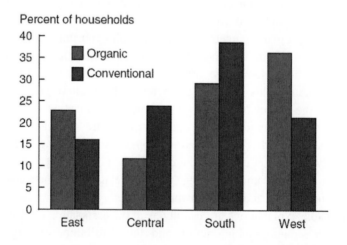

Figure 1. Distribution of organic and conventional milk households by region, 2004.

Percent of households

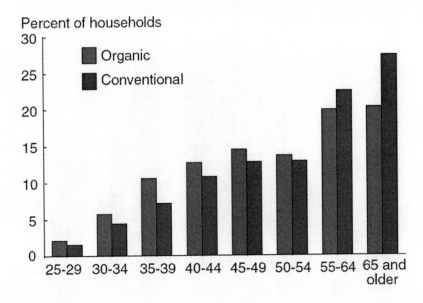

Figure 2. Distribution of organic and conventional milk households by age of head of household, 2004.

Percent of households

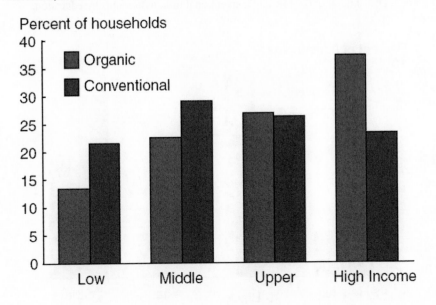

Figure 3. Distribution of organic and conventional milk households by income,**
2004.

Percent of households

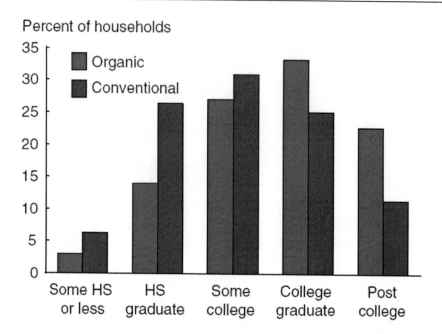

Figure 4. Distribution of organic and conventional milk households by education, 2004.

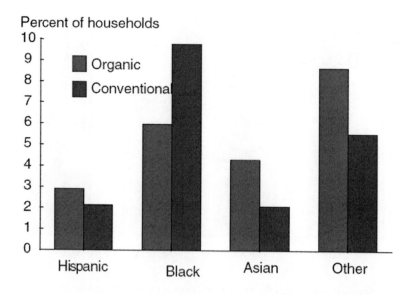

Figure 5. Distribution of organic and conventional milk households by ethnicity,* 2004.

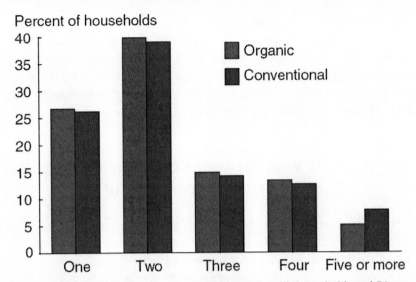

*White households comprise 71 percent of the organic milk households and 74 percent of the conventional milk households and were omitted from figure 5 because their presence overwhelmed the chart.

**See box on page 5 for information on income categories.

Source: Calculated by USDA, ERS from Nielsen data, using the Nielsen projection factor.

Figure 6. Distribution of organic and conventional milk households by household size, 2004.

Few Factors Influence Organic Milk's Average Share of the Milk Budget Of the households that purchase organic milk, the mean share of milk expenditures devoted to organic milk purchases is 32 percent and the median share is 13 percent. The disparity between the mean and the median indicates that some households buy a lot of organic milk and that many households buy a small amount, relative to the total amount of milk purchased. Shares vary less among the households who devote one-third or more of their milk budget toward organic milk: these households are frequent purchasers of organic milk, and 36 percent of the organic households are in this category, with an average expenditure share of 73 percent and a median share of 75 percent.

Once a household has made the decision to purchase organic milk, few demographic factors appear to have a large influence on the average share of milk expenditures allotted to organic milk, or the frequency of organic milk purchases (figure 7). Households with four or more members have a smaller expenditure share than the average household, as do upper income households (those with income between $44,999 and $69,999; see box, "Nielsen Homescan Panel Data" on page 5). Households headed by younger people, those with the highest level of education, Asian and Black households, and households living in the South and Central regions have a higher average expenditure share than the typical organic household. The remaining demographic factors have little if any influence on the average expenditure share.

OLD AND NEW WISDOM ABOUT ORGANIC CONSUMERS: COMPETING OR CONSISTENT IDEAS?

There are several accepted beliefs about the organic sector and the organic consumer. The industry is in a state of transition, as suggested by recent Hartman studies, and is moving or has moved from the old vision of White, well educated, high-income consumers with young children as the main purchasers of organic food to one where lower income people purchase a large share of organic food. Part of the transition focuses on broader ethnic groups as organic food consumers. Simultaneously, conventional supermarkets are selling a large share of organic food, especially for such products as cow milk and soymilk. Some in the industry are concerned that the supply needs of Wal-Mart and other large companies may trigger a shift toward larger organic farms and firms, pressure to weaken the USDA organic standards (see box, "National Organic Standards"), and downward pressure on prices that will reduce domestic producers' profits (Gogoi, 2006; *New York Times*, 2006).

The data in this chapter provide a snapshot of the organic milk market in 2004 and, thus, cannot validate trends in the organic industry or for organic milk specifically (a long enough time series on organic purchases is not yet available to make such a study possible). Yet, the data do provide insight into the market. First, nearly all organic milk is sold in conventional channels, thus indirectly supporting the notion that organic products have been integrated into more traditional market channels as products shift from health food stores to conventional supermarkets. Most organic milk is purchased in conventional supermarkets; in fact, a larger share of organic milk (relative to conventional milk) is purchased in this traditional venue. Compared with conventional milk sales, a far smaller share of organic milk sales takes place in supercenters and mass merchandisers. Second, the 2004 price premiums for organic milk are high, suggesting that increasing presence in the conventional supermarkets has not eliminated price premiums. One factor contributing to these large premiums is the relative scarcity of organic milk. Whether large price premiums continue into the future depends on the interplay among the major retailers, supply from organic dairies, and consumer demand for organic milk.

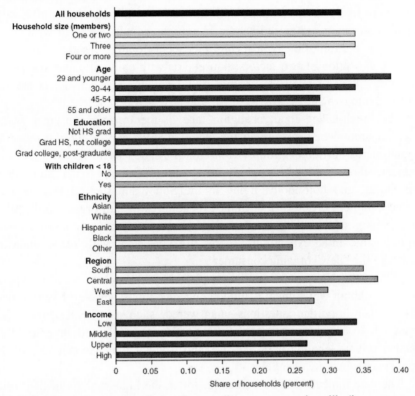

Note: Chart reports average share of expenditures on organic milk (i.e., average of organic share of expenditures, or expenditures on organic milk divided by total milk expenditures) over all organic households in each category.

Source: Calculated by USDA, ERS from Nielsen data, using the Nielsen projection factor.

Figure 7. Share of milk expenditures that are for organic milk, by demographic factor, 2004.

The demographic characteristics of the organic milk consumer in 2004, as revealed by the Nielsen Homescan data, support some—but not all—of the notions about the sector. Data show that the typical consumer of organic milk is White, well educated, and living in a household headed by someone younger than age 50. Households of all income levels purchase organic milk, although

61 percent of the households buying organic milk have annual incomes of at least $50,000. Across ethnic groups or race, a higher share of Asian, Hispanic, and "Other" consumers purchased organic milk rather than conventional milk. Education influences purchases of organic milk: those with higher education were more likely to buy organic milk than those with less education. Lastly, organic consumers are more likely to live on the country's east or west coast. In sum, the portrait of the typical consumer seems to hold, based on these data, with the exception of two factors: households with children under age 18 are not more likely to purchase organic milk,[7] and organic consumers are not clustered into two age groups.

The much-talked-about changing face of the organic consumer seems more apparent when examining the share of milk expenditures devoted to organic across different groups. Households headed by a person age 45 or younger, those with the highest level of education, Asian and Black households, and households living in the South and Central U.S. regions devote a higher portion of their milk expenditures toward organic milk. With the exception of the role of education, these characteristics of consumers with large organic milk expenditure shares are consistent with recent industry studies of the "new" organic consumer.

While the descriptive statistics provide a snapshot of a group of consumers about which there is little knowledge, the reliance on 1 year of data leaves other important questions unanswered, such as whether the USDA organic logo has increased consumer confidence and retail organic sales, whether private labeling is on the rise, and whether the characteristics of the organic consumer are changing.

The data indicate that consumers devoting the highest share of their milk expenditures toward organic milk in 2004 were relatively younger, of diverse ethnicity, and highly educated, in contrast to the organic consumer of the previous decade. Further, households of all income categories and across all ethnic groups are buying organic milk. The variety in the types of consumers buying organic milk suggests that the market continues to expand. The noted supply shortages suggest that there may still be untapped consumer segments for organic milk, and if commercial dairies are successful in producing organic milk at lower prices, new consumers are likely to begin purchasing organic milk. Clearly, opportunities exist for organic dairy producers and conventional producers considering converting their operations to organic production.

REFERENCES

ACNielsen. (2005). *The Power of Private Label 2005: A Review of Growth Trends Around the World.* September. Accessed April 2006 at: http://www2. acnielsen. com/reports/documents/2005_privatelabel.pdf

Barry, M. (2004). "The New World Order: Organic Consumer Lifestyle Segmentation." *[N]sight.* Volume *VI*, Number 2.

Baxter, Brent. (2006). *"who's buying organic?: demographics 2006,"* hartbeat taking the pulse of the marketplace, May 17. Accessed at http://www.hartman-group.com/products/HB/2006_05_17.html; August 3, 2006

Budgar, Laurie. (2006). "Convenience and Health Drive Natural Food Sales." *The Natural Foods Merchandiser.* June.

Demeritt, L. (2004). "Organic Pathways." *[N]Sight.* Hartman Group, Inc. Bellevue, WA.

Glaser, Lewrene K. & Gary Thompson. (2000). *"The Demand for Organic and Conventional Milk."* Presented at the Western Agricultural Economics Association meeting, Vancouver, British Columbia.

Gogoi, P. (2006). "Wal-Mart's Organic Offensive." *Business Week.* March 29.

Hartman Group. 2000. *The Organic Consumer Profile.* Bellevue, WA.

Hartman Group. (2002). *Hartman Organic Research Review: A Compilation of National Organic Research Conducted by the Hartman Group.* Bellevue, Washington.

Hartman Group. (2004). *Organic Food and Beverage Trends.* Bellevue, Washington.

Hochschulverlag AG and der ETH Zürich. pp. 542-545.

Howie, M. (2004). "Research Roots Out Myths Behind Buying Organic Foods." *Feedstuffs.* March 29.

International Trade Centre (ITC). (1999). *Organic Food and Beverages: World Supply and Major European Markets.* ITC/UNCTAD/WTO, Geneva.

Leibtag, Ephraim. (2005). "Where You Shop Matters: Store Formats Drive Variation in Retail Prices." *Amber Waves.* Vol. 3. Issue 5. November. www.ers.usda.gov/amberwaves/ november05/features/ whereyoushop.htm

Lohr, L. & Semali, A. (2000). "Retailer Decision Making in Organic Produce Marketing." In W.J. Florkowski, S.E. Prussia, and R.L. Shewfelt (eds.). *Integrated View of Fruit and Vegetable Quality.* Technomic Pub. Co., Inc., Lancaster, PA. pp. 201-208.

Lohr, L. (2001). "Factors Affecting International Demand and Trade in Organic Food Products." In *Changing Structure of Global Food Consumption and Trade*, A. Regmi (ed.). Agriculture and Trade Report No. WRS01-1. U.S. Department of Agriculture, Economic Research Service. pp. 67-79. www.ers.usda.gov/publications/wrs011/

Miller, James J. & Don P. Blayney. (2006). *Dairy Backgrounder.* Outlook Report No. LDP-M-145-01. U.S. Department of Agriculture, Economic Research Service. July. www.ers.usda.gov/publications/ldp/2006/07jul/ldpm14501/

New York Times. (2006). *"When Wal-Mart Goes Organic."* Editorial, May 14.

Nutrition Business Journal (NBJ). (2004). *NBJ's Organic Foods Report 2004*, Penton Media, Inc.

Nutrition Business Journal (NBJ). (2006). *U.S. Organic Food Sales ($Mil) 1997-2010e-Chart 22.* Penton Media, Inc.

Oliver, Hilary. (2006). "Organic Dairy Demand Exceeds Supply." *Natural Foods Merchandiser.* August.

Onazaka, Yuko, David Bunch & Douglas Larson. (2006). "What Exactly Are They Paying For? Explaining the Price Premium for Organic Produce." *Agricultural and Resource Economics Update.* Vol. *9*, No. 6. University of California Giannini Foundation. July/August.

Organic Trade Association (OTA). (2006). *Organic Trade Association's 2006 Manufacturer's Survey.* Produced by the Nutrition Business Journal. Greenfield, MA.

Richter, T., Schmid, O., Freyer, B., Halpin, D. & Vetter, R. (2000). "Organic Consumer in Supermarkets – New Consumer Group With Different Buying Behavior and Demands!" In *Proceedings 13th IFOAM Scientific Conference*, T. Alfödi, W. Lockeretz, U. Niggli (eds.). vdf

Thompson, G.D. (1998). "Consumer Demand for Organic Foods: What We Know and What We Need to Know." *American Journal of Agricultural Economics*, 80, 1113-1118.

U.S. Department of Agriculture. (2002a). *Organic Food Standards and Their Labels: The Facts.* National Organic Program, April 2002, updated January 2007. Accessed February 7, 2007, at http://www.ams.usda.gov/nop/consumers/brochure.html

U.S. Department of Agriculture. (2002b). *Background Information.* National Organic Program, October 2002, updated January 2007. Accessed April 30, 2007, at http://www.ams.usda.gov/nop/ FactSheets/Backgrounder.html

Wal-Mart. (2006). "Organics for Everyone." Accessed August 2006 at http://walmart.triaddigital.com/OrganicsContent.aspx?c=Organics+For+E veryone&s=Wal-mart

Weinraub, J. & W. Nicholls. (2005). "Organic Milk Supply Falls Short." *Washington Post*. June 1. pg. F01.

Whole Foods Market. (2005). *"Nearly Two-Thirds of Americans Have Tried Organic Foods and Beverages."* Accessed August 2006 at http://www.whole foodsmarket.com/company/pr_11-18-05.html

End Notes

[1] The 6-percent estimate is based on 2005 total milk retail sales of approximately $17 billion, as estimated by ERS. The *Nutrition Business Journal* reports retail sales of organic milk/cream, not just organic milk; the share of organic milk is less than 6 percent.

[2] Supply responses necessarily lag behind increases in consumer demand because it takes 3 years to convert farmland to meet organic standards so that they can provide organic feed. The cows have to be managed organically and fed organic feed for 1 year. But under a special provision passed into law in 2006, dairies that are converting to organic can convert their farmland and pastures for 2 years and then use the feed and pasture raised during the last year of conversion to the converting cows. That way, the farm and the cows all finish conversion together.

[3] Distribution of organic food by market channel is only available for 2003 and 2005. We chose to use the most recent data in table 1 (2005).

[4] The Nielsen data report the name of the store where each purchase was made; the most easily identifiable natural products grocery venues are Whole Foods, Wild Oats, and health food stores labeled "Other—health food store."

[5] Most organic milk is sold by the half gallon, while most conventional milk is sold by the quart or the gallon. Because of the presence of the measure in the organic market, we decided to use the half-gallon price as the basis for this analysis.

[6] According to the National Organic Program, organic food is produced by farmers who emphasize the use of renewable resources and the conservation of soil and water to enhance environmental quality for future generations (USDA, 2002b).

[7] The accepted notion is that households with young children buy more organic food. This analysis used children under age 18 rather than young children, and so does not exactly examine the accepted wisdom.

INDEX